Dyslexia and mathematics

Edited by
T.R. and E. Miles

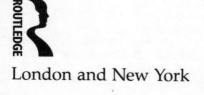

London and New York

First published 1992
by Routledge
11 New Fetter Lane, London EC4P 4EE

Simultaneously published in the USA and Canada
by Routledge
a division of Routledge, Chapman and Hall, Inc.
29 West 35th Street, New York, NY 10001

© 1992 T.R. Miles and E. Miles

Typeset in Parlament by
Leaper & Gard Ltd, Bristol
Printed and bound in Great Britain by
Biddles Ltd, Guildford and King's Lynn

British Library Cataloguing in Publication Data
Dyslexia and Mathematics.
  1. Dyslexic children. Education. Curriculum, mathematics
  I. Miles, T. R. (Thomas Richard) 1923–   II. Miles, Elaine
  371.9144

  ISBN 0–415–06480–5
  ISBN 0–415–04987–3 (pbk)

Library of Congress Cataloging in Publication Data
Dyslexia and Mathematics/Edited by T.R. and E. Miles
  Includes bibliographical references and indexes.
  ISBN 0–415–06480–5 – ISBN 0–415–04987–3 (pbk)
  1. Mathematics–Study and teaching.   2. Dyslexic children–
  Education.   I. Miles, T. R. (Thomas Richard)   II. Miles, Elaine.
  QA11.D97   1991
  371.91'44—dc20

Contents

Figures and tables

Figures

Tables

Contributors

J.R. Ashcroft (BSc) is Deputy Headmaster and Head of Mathematics at Mark College, Mark, Highbridge, Somerset.

S.J. Chinn (BSc, PhD, Dip. Ed. Man., PGCE) is Headmaster of Mark College, Mark, Highbridge, Somerset.

Anne Henderson (B.Ed.) lectures for the Dyslexia Unit, University College of North Wales, Bangor, and is a teacher at St. David's College, Llandudno.

Mary Kibel (BA, PGCE) runs a workshop in Exeter for the Devon Dyslexia Association and is a 'special needs' teacher in the county of Devon.

Elaine Miles (MA, Dip. Ed.) is in charge of courses for teachers of dyslexic children at the Dyslexia Unit, University College of North Wales, Bangor.

T.R. Miles (MA, PhD, C. Psychol., FBPsS) is Professor Emeritus of Psychology at the University College of North Wales, Bangor.

Preface

The central theme of this book is that the difficulties experienced by dyslexics in mathematics are manifestations of the same limitation which also affects their reading and spelling. From this it follows that the appropriate teaching techniques are likely to involve the same basic principles. In the words of Ansara (1973: 120): 'The insights the therapist brings to the teaching of language skills to a dyslexic student may be especially helpful in the teaching of basic mathematics.'

Now, as far as language skills are concerned, the practical experiences of specialist teachers of dyslexics over many years, coupled, more recently, with telling research evidence, leave little doubt as to what the basic principles of teaching should be. Systematic programmes are available, in particular those written by Gillingham and Stillman (1969), Hornsby and Shear (1975), Hickey (1977) and E. Miles (1989). In the case of mathematics, however, the situation is different. In the first place there is no comparable body of expertise either of research or of teaching experience; second, mathematics is a vast subject, and it would therefore be no easy matter to determine what should be the priorities as regards topics to be taught.

For these reasons it seemed to us that it would be premature to try to produce a kind of Gillingham–Stillman manual for the teaching of mathematics. Instead we thought it would be preferable to produce an edited book in which different contributors could write on the subject of 'dyslexia and mathematics' from their personal point of view. Besides setting out some of our own ideas, we wished, in particular, to draw on the experience of those who were currently teaching mathematics to dyslexics but who over many years had taught them literacy skills and were interested in the theoretical relationships between the two. Our intention was to give the reader, not, of course, a structured programme or a summary of conclusively established research findings, but rather some suggested ways forward which we hoped would eventually lead both to improved practice and to greater theoretical understanding. It gave us great pleasure when the four people whom we approached all agreed to contribute.

Finally, to avoid any possible misunderstanding, we should like to make clear that this is a book about dyslexia (or, strictly, specific developmental dyslexia), not about 'good practice' in teaching mathematics in general. Our purpose is to demonstrate the usefulness of the dyslexia concept in the area of mathematics, and no concessions are made to those who question its usefulness even in the area of literacy. We do not, of course, dispute that some of the procedures advocated may be of help to non-dyslexics as well as to dyslexics (as, indeed, some of our contributors make clear). The reason for this is simply that techniques which are essential for those who have a specific limitation are likely, at the very least, to be helpful to those who do not; and it is certainly not being claimed that the kinds of mistake which are made by dyslexics are never made by anyone else! To put the matter another way, if there is bad practice it seems likely that intelligent non-dyslexics may in many cases survive it without any major disaster, whereas its effect even on the most intelligent dyslexics is likely to be catastrophic. It is also important to recognize that there are some aspects of mathematics, for example, recognition of patterns, which the typical dyslexic seldom finds difficult. In·all these respects, therefore, the mathematical needs of dyslexics are distinctive, and the present book was written with these needs in mind.

T.R.M.
E.M.
Bangor

REFERENCES

Ansara, A. (1973) 'The language therapist as a basic mathematics tutor for adolescents', *Bulletin of the Orton Society* 23, 119–39.

Gillingham, A. and Stillman, B.E. (1969) *Remedial Training for Children with Specific Disability in Reading, Spelling and Penmanship*, Cambridge, Mass., Educators Publishing Service.

Hickey, K. (1977) *A Language Training Course for Teachers and Learners*, Wimbledon, London, Elizabeth Adams Publications.

Hornsby, B. and Shear, F. (1975) *Alpha to Omega,* London, Heinemann
    Educational Books.
Miles, E. (1989) *The Bangor Dyslexia Teaching System,* London: Whurr.

Conventions

To avoid ugly circumlocutions we have referred, other things being equal, to the teacher as 'she' and to the pupil as 'he'. We take it as obvious that both teachers and pupils can be of either sex!

Chapter 1

Some theoretical considerations

T.R. Miles

THE NATURE OF DYSLEXIA

Descriptions of children who would now be called 'dyslexic' go back almost 100 years. Those who have written on the subject include Morgan (1896), Hinshelwood (1917), Orton (1937), MacMeeken (1939), Hallgren (1950), Hermann (1959), Critchley (1970), Naidoo (1972), Critchley and Critchley (1978), Vellutino (1979), Miles (1983, 1987), Thomson (1984), Snowling (1987), Kamhi and Catts (1989) and Miles and Miles (1990). Some of the more important indications of dyslexia include lateness in learning to read, relatively weak spelling even after many hours of tuition, weak memory for disconnected items in series, such as the months of the year or visually or auditorily presented digits, and uncertainty over left and right. Above all, the teacher or parent is left with a sense of incongruity: despite their literacy problems dyslexics may show considerable ability in certain areas, for instance in the recognizing of logical relationships, in art and modelling, and in mechanical and engineering tasks. Dyslexia can usefully be described as a 'syndrome' – that is, a pattern of signs which regularly go together: any one of these signs on its own would be of no special significance, but if several of them co-occur in the same individual they take on a meaning which none of them would have had in isolation.

There is good reason for believing that the difficulties of the dyslexic have a physical basis. The earliest investigators, Morgan, Hinshelwood and Orton, were quick to point out the similarities between children showing these developmental anomalies and adults whose language skills were affected because of acquired injury. It also became plain that the difficulties could occur in individuals whose backgrounds were widely different, and it became virtually impossible to invoke either of the once-fashionable scapegoats, poor teaching and over-anxiety in the parents, as the main causal factor. It is known that dyslexia occurs more frequently in boys than in girls (Finucci and Childs 1981), and it is also known that a genetic factor is often involved (Hallgren 1950; Finucci *et al.* 1976; DeFries *et al.* 1987). Finally, there is evidence based on postmortem examination of the brains of individuals who had been reliably diagnosed as dyslexic in their lifetime. According to a recently published report (Galaburda 1989), eight brains have so far been examined, six male, two female. Particular attention has been paid to the *planum temporale* which forms part of the temporal lobe. It had already been established, some two decades earlier, that the *plana* in the two cerebral hemispheres are asymmetrical in about 75 per cent of cases. In none of the dyslexic brains, however, was this asymmetry present; and that this should have happened, with no exceptions, in eight consecutive cases is clearly a finding of major significance. In addition, all eight brains showed structural abnormalities, including ectopias (intrusions of cells from one layer to another) and dysplasias (disorganizations of cells within a cell layer). Galaburda and his colleagues have been cautious in interpreting these findings. One possibility, however, is that the balance between the two cerebral hemispheres is different in dyslexics and that this leads to relative difficulties in the processing of symbolic or linguistic material (usually a function of the left hemisphere) and to relative strength at so-called 'right hemisphere' tasks, namely, those which involve spatial awareness or overall planning. This hypothesis, though not conclusively established, at least makes sense of much that would otherwise be puzzling about dyslexics' observed behaviour.

There is evidence from cognitive psychology that all or most dyslexics have difficulty at the phonological level, where 'phonology' is the science of speech sounds in so far as they convey meaning. (For a review of the evidence in this area see Catts 1989.) Vellutino (1987) speaks in this connection of 'the inability to represent and access the sound of a word in order to help remember the word'.

One could also characterize the dyslexic's difficulty as a weakness at 'paired associate learning' – though with the proviso that this applies not to the learning of all associations but only to those which involve the understanding of symbols. In traditional experiments with humans the subjects are given a stimulus which is 'paired' with another stimulus. For example, a nonsense shape presented visually is paired with its 'name', that is a nonsense word presented auditorily; and after the name has been supplied on a number of occasions the subjects are eventually able to say it correctly as soon as the visual stimulus is exposed. Their performance is scored by noting how many times they have to be supplied with the correct name before they can produce it without any prompting. There is evidence (Done and Miles 1978) which suggests that dyslexics may require more 'pairings' in such a task than do non-dyslexics. Moreover, even when the requisite associations have been formed, it has been found that the response latency, that is, the time needed to produce the right word, tends to be longer in the case of dyslexics than in the case of non-dyslexics (Spring and Capps 1974; Done and Miles 1988). This limitation has repercussions on the ability to notice detail, for example the exact letters needed for the spelling of a word, since fewer letters can be named per unit time. It also makes sense of the relative weakness of dyslexics at tasks involving immediate memory, such as the recall of auditorily or visually presented digits (Rugel 1974; Ellis and Miles 1977; Miles 1983).

In contrast, dyslexics have been found to be strong at a variety of other tasks, for example, the ability to pick out similarities and recognize relationships. Steeves (1983) reports that some of her dyslexic subjects obtained very high scores on the Standard Progressive Matrices (SPM) (Raven 1958), while Miles (1983, 1987) reports similar successes on the Advanced Matrices (Raven 1965). In the case of the 'Similarities' item ('How are ... and ... alike?'), which occurs in the Wechsler Intelligence Scale for Children (Wechsler 1969), the evidence suggests that dyslexic children are not normally disadvantaged (Rugel 1974; Spache 1976; Miles and Ellis 1981), while in the case of the corresponding item in the British Ability Scales (Elliott et al. 1979), Thomson (1982) found that dyslexics at three different age levels (9.0 to 9.11, 10.0 to 10.11, and 11.0 to 11.11) were consistently able to score highly.

In a somewhat speculative paper Ellis and Miles (1981) drew a distinction between the 'lexical' system and the 'semantic' system. The model used was that of an internal 'dictionary' (or 'lexicon'): learning to talk was envisaged as a process of building up entries in the lexicon while use of the correct word was assumed to involve retrieval from it. In contrast, the semantic system was postulated as a device which was responsible for processing for meaning. Identification of letters was therefore primarily a lexical task, while the recognition of similarities was primarily a semantic one. Since the two systems were assumed to be separate it was possible on their view for the same individual to be strong at tasks involving the one and weak at tasks involving the other. This they believe to be true in the case of dyslexics: on their view it makes sense of the reported evidence on dyslexia if one assumes a deficit on the lexical side but no distinctive problems on the semantic side. Since this distinction may contribute to our understanding of dyslexics' mathematical strengths and weaknesses, it will be taken up in the next section.

THE PERFORMANCE OF DYSLEXICS AT MATHEMATICS

What, then, are the mathematical strengths and weaknesses of typical dyslexics and how might one make sense of them in the light of the above theory?

The evidence in this area is somewhat limited. A computer search based on the word 'dyslexia' and going back as far as 1966 disclosed only very few papers in the area of dyslexia and mathematics. There is, of course, a massive literature on mathematical difficulties in general, but valuable though many of these studies are relatively few of the writers refer to dyslexia as such or describe children who are recognizably dyslexic, while fewer still have carried out controlled studies comparing dyslexics with non-dyslexics. In these circumstances it seemed to me that the most helpful way of proceeding would be to draw on such sources as are available and to indicate the position as I myself see it, while at the same time giving readers the chance to evaluate the evidence for themselves. I have therefore grouped this evidence under three heads, namely, (a) controlled comparisons, (b) results of intelligence test scores, and (c) clinical and individual observations. Although controlled comparisons can rightly be regarded as the most telling form of evidence (provided the research has been adequately designed), it by no means follows that other observations can simply be dismissed, particularly if a coherent picture emerges overall, which I believe it does.

Controlled comparisons

One of the most important of these comparisons was that carried out by Steeves (1983). Her subjects were 54 dyslexic boys between the ages of 10 and 14 years and 54 suitably-matched controls. She divided them into four groups, namely (i) 'dyslexics high' (DH), that is, dyslexics with a high score on the SPM test (Raven 1958), (ii) 'dyslexics average' (DA), that is, dyslexics with an average score on the SPM, (iii) non-dyslexics in an advanced (or 'high') class for mathematics (NH), and (iv) non-dyslexics in an average class for mathematics (NA). The DH group were found on testing to be at the same level as the NH group on the SPM; on a test of school mathematics, however, they scored lower than the NH group and were on a level with the NA group, while on the Wechsler Memory Test they scored lower than both the non-dyslexic groups. The DA group were on a level with the NA group on the SPM but below them on the other two tests, being particularly weak on the Wechsler Memory Test.

On the basis of these results Steeves is in no doubt that some dyslexics can be gifted mathematically, and, indeed, if this were not so, it is hard to see how the DH group could have been on a level with an 'average' group of non-dyslexics on a school mathematics test. Since, however, a high score on the SPM is widely agreed to constitute evidence for mathematical potential, the question arises as to why the DH group scored lower than the NH group on the mathematics test. Now Steeves convincingly argues that, since they scored highly on the SPM, any weaknesses that they showed could not have been due to lack of maturity, visual weakness, spatial problems, perceptual confusion, or sequencing difficulties. Where they in fact came down was on the Wechsler Memory Test – and here they obtained lower scores than even the NA group, despite their higher scores on the SPM. Her suggested explanation – which is coherent with what is known about dyslexia from other sources – is that, despite their high potential, they were handicapped at mathematics by those parts of the subject which call for memorizing ability. She does not suggest in detail what part is played by this memory limitation. There is evidence from other research, however, that, as far as mathematics is concerned, a weakness at immediate recall of number facts may be one of the limitations. This is the issue to which we must now turn.

In a study by Ackerman *et al.* (1986) the subjects were (among others) 24 'reading disabled' children and 24 controls. All were given sums of varying degrees of complexity and were asked, in timed conditions, to judge whether the solution given was true or false. On the basis of the results they were assigned to one of four categories, namely, 'fast and accurate', 'slow and accurate', 'fast and inaccurate', and 'slow and inaccurate'. Sixteen of the 'reading disabled' group were 'slow and inaccurate' while 20 out of the 24 controls were 'fast and accurate'. On the assumption that all or most of the 'reading disabled' children were in fact dyslexic, these findings suggest that dyslexics may tend to have fewer number facts available for immediate use, or, in the authors' words, have not yet achieved 'automatization'.

In a study carried out by Fleischner et al. (1982), written tests of addition, subtraction and multiplication were given in timed conditions to 183 'learning disabled' children and 842 controls. The former were found to be both slower and less accurate. Although there are possible difficulties in the interpretation of these results (not all the 'learning disabled' group were necessarily dyslexic in the required sense and there was no strict matching for intelligence), there is at least evidence – in the authors' words – that 'the LD children in this study were not so proficient in basic fact calculation as their nondisabled peers' (ibid.: 54).

In a further study (Pritchard et al. 1989) the subjects (15 dyslexic boys aged 12 to 14 and 15 age-matched controls) were given multiplication sums involving all the 'times tables' up to 16. They were asked to say whether they could give the answer and, if so, whether they knew it 'in one' or had to work it out. One point was awarded for every product known 'in one'. Almost without exception the dyslexics had fewer number facts available than the controls, though the differences were less marked in the case of the $5\times$, $10\times$, and $11\times$ tables. The authors suggest that in the case of these three tables dyslexics are able to some extent to compensate for their limited knowledge of number facts by making use of the regular patterning. They also point out that there is one basic regularity in the number system which can be used if all else fails, viz. that *the numbers go up in ones*. They tentatively suggest that the reason why many dyslexics use their fingers or put marks on paper when doing calculations is because the requisite number fact is not immediately available to them by any other means. It is thus a typically dyslexic 'compensatory strategy'.

In this connection Ashcraft and Fierman (1982) have distinguished 'counting' from 'memory retrieval'. When children aged 9 and upwards (grades 3, 4, and 6) were presented with addition sums and had to say if the answer given was 'true' or 'false', there appeared to be differences in their processing procedures at different ages. 'Reaction time patterns suggested that third grade is a transitional stage with respect to memory structure for addition – half of these children seemed to be counting and half retrieving from memory' (ibid.: 216). It may be surmised from this finding that dyslexics, if they make the transition at all, do not do so until a somewhat later age.

The claim that poor memory and weakness at mathematics are associated finds further support from a study by Webster (1979). In this study the subjects were 73 sixth grade children who were within the average range on the Peabody Picture Vocabulary Test (PPVT): 24 were 'mildly disabled' at mathematics (as judged by the arithmetic sub-test of the Wide Range Achievement Test), 26 were 'severely disabled', while 23, serving as controls, were at grade level or higher. All subjects were required to recall strings of seven non-rhyming consonants and strings of seven digits. Each stimulus was presented for 1 second with a 1 second interval between each presentation; and by a suitable statistical technique the influence of intelligence, as judged by scores on the PPVT, was kept constant. The general trend was clear: in both visual and auditory conditions the controls remembered more than those in the 'mildly disabled' group and more still than those in the 'severely disabled' group. A likely interpretation seems to be that an adequate immediate memory is a necessary condition for mathematical progress; and since dyslexics are known to be weak in this area (see p. 1) their weakness at mathematics would in that case not be at all surprising.

Miles (1983) has reported that, in a sample of 132 dyslexics, 90 per cent of those aged 7 and 8, 96 per cent of those aged 9, 10, 11, and 12, and 85 per cent of those aged 13 to 18 had difficulties of one kind or another in reciting the 6×, 7×, and 8× tables; the corresponding percentages for suitably matched non-dyslexics were 71, 51, and 53. In the case of a series of six subtraction items of varying difficulty ($9 - 2$, $19 - 7$, $52 - 9$, and so on) the percentages were 86, 58, and 63 for the dyslexics, compared with 62, 19, and 10 for the controls. These findings suggest that some dyslexics remain weak at subtraction and that the great majority have distinctive problems with tables. This issue will be discussed further on pp. 12–15.

Finally, as part of a series of very interesting enquiries into dyslexia and mathematics, Joffe (1981) gave a test of computation to 51 dyslexics, aged between 8 and 17, and to a similar number of controls. All the subjects had been found to be of average intelligence or above on standardized tests, and the dyslexics had been diagnosed as such at the University of Aston. When the test results for the different ages were combined she found that about 10 per cent of the dyslexics scored very highly, whereas about 60 per cent scored well below expectation.

This finding confirms the view that some dyslexics can be extremely successful mathematicians – a conclusion which is in line both with the claims of Steeves (see above) and with the informal evidence which will be cited on pp. 11–16. Overall, Joffe has reached a position with regard to dyslexia and mathematics which is basically similar to that adopted in the present book. For example, in a later paper (Joffe 1983) she writes as follows:

> Historically, dyslexia has been seen in terms of difficulties relating to reading and spelling.... But limiting the features of dyslexia in this way is tantamount to ignoring the full story – it is putting the cart before the horse; looking at external manifestations of the difficulty while largely ignoring its origin and the implications of its aetiology.... If one is talking about dyslexia one is talking about a constellation of difficulties.... It is clear that written language and school mathematics share a lot of common features.

There is one possible criticism, however, viz. that she has made too much of the figures of 60 and 40 per cent. In her own words (Joffe 1990):

> Happily, about 10 per cent of dyslexics are likely to be really successful in mathematics and about 30 per cent exhibit no particular difficulty, so it is just the 60 per cent you have to worry about.

The inference, however, that 40 per cent of dyslexics can do mathematics and that 60 per cent have a problem seems simplistic; in particular it does not do justice to the complexity of the facts as reported by Steeves. It is possible, in particular, that Joffe's figures of 60 and 40 per cent conceal the fact that some of the 60 per cent had strengths and some of the 40 per cent had weaknesses. An alternative explanation, equally compatible with Joffe's data as presented, is that *all* dyslexics have difficulties of some kind with mathematics (as part and parcel of their problems with language and memory) but that there is considerable variation in the extent to which these difficulties are overcome. It might have been found, for instance, that some of the 40 per cent would have stumbled if they had been asked to recite the 6×, 7× and 8× tables, as they were in the Miles (1983) study. Moreover, since it is agreed that dyslexics cannot easily recall strings of digits, whether presented auditorily or visually, it is surely possible that at least some of the 40 per cent would have had difficulty in adding up columns of figures. Despite the value of Joffe's research in general, therefore, the use which she makes of these percentages seems somewhat questionable.

Results of intelligence test scores

There are good grounds for believing that a significant number of poor readers (whatever the precise criteria by which they were picked out) obtain relatively low scores in the arithmetic sub-test of the Wechsler Intelligence Scale for Children (WISC) (Wechsler 1969). The so-called ACID profile (weakness at the Arithmetic, Coding, Information and Digit Span sub-tests) is now a well-established phenomenon (Rugel 1974; Spache 1976; Naidoo 1972; Richards 1985); and it has been argued by Miles and Ellis (1981) that the lexical deficiency hypothesis makes sense of these distinctive weaknesses. So far, however, the analysis of WISC sub-test scores has been only coarse grained; and in the case of the Arithmetic sub-test in particular it would, I think, be informative to analyse in detail what is involved in the different items and compare the performance of individual children. Since the items are read orally (one repetition is allowed) there may be memory problems; and because there are time limits for each answer those who process information slowly may be at a disadvantage, the more so since no extra time allowance is given if the question has to be repeated. Any child, including a dyslexic, who has learned the names of the numbers and has grasped how the number system works will almost certainly be able to do the first seven items. Most of the items from 10 onwards, however, require a knowledge of tables – something at which dyslexics are known to be weak (Miles 1983). Much, therefore, will depend on the number and nature of the compensatory strategies that the child has been able to acquire, either by himself or with the assistance of parents and teachers.

Now because the items have been carefully arranged in order of difficulty it follows that a young dyslexic, aged, say, 7 or 8, unless he is very precocious, is not expected to succeed beyond a certain point; and this means that his distinctive weaknesses (over tables, and so on) will not have been exposed. As a result, his score is likely to be within normal limits, even though the scores for older dyslexics may be depressed. Thus if results for dyslexic children of different ages are combined there may well be evidence of a trend but one would not expect it to be a very pronounced one; and there is the further complication that some dyslexics will have overcome their initial limitation more than others. It seems fair to conclude that a score on the WISC Arithmetic sub-test, unless it is accompanied by detailed item analysis, will be of little diagnostic value in the case of a dyslexic since it may represent a kind of compromise between his high reasoning ability and his typical dyslexic weaknesses. As will be pointed out by Dr Chinn in Chapter 2, the result of any test of mathematics is liable to be misleading if one takes into account only the score and fails to take account of the way in which the subject reached his answer.

The same arguments hold in the case of the Basic Arithmetic item in the British Ability Scales (BAS) (Elliott et al. 1979). As part of his study of the performance of dyslexics on the BAS, Thomson (1982) showed that dyslexics in three different age groups (8 to 10, 11 to 13, and 14 to 16) scored consistently lower on this item than they did on certain others such as Similarities, Matrices and Visualization of Cubes.

The variety of results when dyslexics are given tests in mathematics is something which any theory of dyslexia has to take into account; and a possible explanation is that a constitutionally based weak lexical system plays an initial causal role, but that, as a result of individual differences in the power of the semantic system and in the teaching to which the child is exposed, the range of scores is extremely wide.

Further evidence from the results of intelligence tests, in the form of individual observations, will be presented in the next section.

Clinical and individual observations

This section will be concerned with evidence based on clinical studies and individual reports.

There is relatively little in the earlier dyslexia literature on mathematical difficulties. Critchley (1970: 45), for example, takes the view that 'arithmetical retardation may be associated with developmental dyslexia, but not necessarily so'. He does, however, give examples of three dyslexics who showed confusion over place value, for instance by writing the wrong number of noughts or by putting the commas in the wrong place. In general, however, his emphasis is on the variety found in dyslexics. There may be:

> an inability to visualize numbers, to memorize the multiplication tables, or to retain a series of digits in the memory for a sufficient time. But in some cases at least, 'mental arithmetic' is carried out with fair success. . . . It is as though they were more at ease upon levels of high abstraction than with verbal symbols. . . . In my experience of dyslexics, however, above-average attainment in mathematics has been rare.
>
> (Ibid.: 48)

Subsequent evidence, however, has established beyond doubt that high level success in mathematics is at least *possible*. It is perhaps wise to treat with caution the claim that Einstein was dyslexic, since although one regularly finds it in the dyslexia literature, the evidence is at best incomplete. Even if this claim is discounted, however, there is hard evidence in relation to other individuals. In particular Jansons (1988), who is now a university lecturer in mathematics, has given a personal account of how he was able to cope with his dyslexic problems.

The overall evidence suggests that all or most dyslexics do, indeed, have difficulty with some aspects of mathematics, but that in spite of this a high level of success is possible. Thus Griffiths (1980: 50–3) cites the case of a university lecturer in physics who in middle age was still found to be insecure on his 6× table. Steeves (1983: 141) cites the case of a 9-year-old dyslexic boy who had been given some graph paper and who after no more than 12 seconds 'called out excitedly that there were 28,000 little squares on his sheet of paper'. Yet this boy had been found to be two years below grade level at reading and spelling and had come out as only average on an arithmetic test.

In addition, Miles (1983) has given many examples of dyslexics with obvious mathematical ability who nevertheless had difficulty with addition and subtraction. His account of the matter is as follows (ibid.: 120–1):

In a number of cases I have seen complex reasoning co-existing with elementary difficulties over calculation. Thus it was plain, in the Terman Merrill cans-of-water item that S 109 was fully clear as to the kind of solution that was needed, but only after careful working out was he able to discover that 9 + 4 = 13! Similarly S 201, when given the Terman Merrill 'tree' item, produced some fully coherent arguments, marred only by the fact that he believed the difference between 18 and 27 to be 11. . . . When one looks at the attempts of dyslexic subjects to do subtraction and addition, the overall picture is often that of a highly sophisticated person, well capable of quite complex logical reasoning, who is nevertheless severely restricted in his ability to give instant answers, and who therefore has to resort to strategies – often of his own devising – which are time-consuming and may sometimes involve considerable risk of error.

The references in this quotation are to the Stanford-Binet intelligence test (Terman and Merrill 1960), while 'S 109' is a way of referring to a particular subject, all subjects having been given individual numbers. In the relevant 'cans-of-water' item the subject is asked how he would bring back 13 pints of water using a 5-pint can and a 9-pint can, given that he must begin by filling the 9-pint can. In the 'tree' item, which is set at the top grade of 'Superior Adult', the subject is told the height of a tree at the time of planting and at yearly intervals for the next three years. He is then required to work out its height at the end of the fourth year. The problem can be solved by recognizing either an arithmetical or a geometric progression; either way it involves implicit recognition of the concept of 'acceleration'. A further example (Miles 1987: 137) is of an undergraduate student who successfully achieved a degree which required a considerable knowledge of statistics. She reported that she did not know immediately that 6 added to 7 was 13 but 'had a strategy for working it out'.

There is also evidence that dyslexics respond in unusual ways when asked to say their 'times tables'. Miles (1982) has attempted to specify some of these ways and has devised a suitable scoring system. He has concentrated primarily on the 6×, 7× and 8× tables on the grounds that these are the hardest to learn and, unlike the 5×, 9×, 10× and 11×, require memorization rather than the following of a rule. A variety of responses can be scored as 'dyslexia positive'. These include not only errors but any one of the following: loss of place (as exemplified by questions such as 'Was it six sevens I was up to?'), a request to leave out the 'preamble' ('Can I just say "six", "twelve", "eighteen"?') when correct recitation requires 'one six is ...', 'two sixes are ...', and so on), any 'consistent' error (for instance moving from 'six threes are twenty' to 'seven threes are twenty-three'), and any change into the 'wrong' table (for instance, in saying the 6×, 'six sevens are forty-two, six eights are forty-eight, eight eights are sixty-four'). Minor signs, any *two* of which in combination are scored as 'dyslexia positive', include: an attempt to 'reorientate' by going back to a previous product which is known for certain ('epanalepsis') (for instance, 'four sixes are twenty-four, five sixes are ... mm ... let me see, four sixes are twenty-four, five sixes are thirty'), slips and corrections (for instance, 'eight eighties – I mean eight eights') and 'skipping' (for instance passing directly from 'six eights are forty-eight' to 'eight eights are sixty-four'). What is of particular interest is that dyslexics are clearly *vulnerable* when they recite their tables, and it seems likely that the slips and corrections arise because they find themselves under pressure.

There are various ways of making sense of the dyslexic's difficulty over tables. Lack of 'automatization' (Ackerman *et al.* 1986, see above) appears to be one factor in the situation. Thus a subject who makes a 'consistent' error (by passing, say, from $6 \times 3 = 20$ to $7 \times 3 = 23$) clearly does not know 'in one' that $7 \times 3 = 21$. Similarly a subject who knows 'in one', for instance, that $8 \times 7 = 56$ will be in little danger of 'losing the place', whereas if he is hurriedly adding on seven to the previous product the risk is much greater.

Somewhat more speculatively one might argue that automatization can take place only if two numbers have been 'paired' with their product on a sufficient number of occasions. On the hypothesis, then, that dyslexics need more 'pairings' than non-dyslexics, the likelihood will be that with commonly occurring products, for instance those of the 2× table, automatization may be acquired without too much difficulty. In 'intermediate' cases, for instance 8×7, the odds are that almost all non-dyslexics will have achieved automatization whereas many dyslexics will not, while, finally, products such as 43×87 are not automatically known even in the case of non-dyslexics. It is worth noting that in the study by Pritchard *et al.* (1989) it was found that the dyslexics had most number facts available in the case of the 2×, 5×, 10× and 11×. Their relative success at the 2× could perhaps be explained in terms of familiarity, whereas in the case of the other three it seems likely, as was noted earlier, that regularity played an important part. More speculatively, it is possible that in these cases knowledge of the algorithm provides the opportunity for self-instruction and therefore for sub-vocal pairing. This would mean that fresh exposures to, say, '$10 \times 8 = 80$' would not 'pass the child by' in the way in which, for instance, a conversation in a totally foreign language passes us by. The analogy is rather with someone whose knowledge of a language has reached a sufficient level to enable her to benefit from being exposed to that language. In general, dyslexics need more 'exposures' before their responses become automatic.

It may also be of help to think in terms of the building up of lexical entries. If a response has become automatized, this means in effect that there is immediate access to the appropriate entry. The ability to respond 'in one' to a mathematical sum is in that case similar to the ability to recognize a word or phrase 'in one' when reading or to set it down with no hesitation when writing. In the same way having to work out a product (for example, $9 \times 8 = 10 \times 8 - 8 = 80 - 8 = 72$) is like having to deduce a word from its component letters; both are examples of a 'fall back' strategy for use when immediate responding is not possible. In the case of both literacy and numeracy it is, of course, a great advantage in the long run if a large amount of automaticity can be achieved, but it is important in both cases that alternative procedures should be available for use where necessary.

Mention has already been made of the tendency on the part of dyslexics to lose the place when reciting tables. This 'losing the place' can occur in other situations also, in particular when the dyslexic has to add up a column of figures. The following example (hitherto unpublished) relates to a dyslexic business man who was involved with the selling of meat and groceries. When he needed to add up the prices of items which he had sold he started – as anyone else would – by putting the individual items in a vertical column:

    7
    3
   12
   22
   43
   37

Whereas many of us, however, would next sum the right-hand column and arrive at the figure of 24, would carry 2 and then sum the left-hand column, he proceeded to group the numbers in pairs and write down the sum of each pair in a further column. When the operation was complete his sheet of paper looked like this:

```
  7
  3            10
 ___
 12
 22            34
 ___
 43
 37            80
 ___

              124
```

This procedure saved him from ever having to hold in mind more than three figures at a time.

There is also evidence that the difficulties experienced by dyslexics over 'left' and 'right' 'spill over' into mathematics. A tiresome complication is that, of the four basic operations, three of them (addition, subtraction and multiplication) require to be started on the right, whereas division has to be started on the left – as does writing across the page. Now unless dyslexics have an adequate understanding as to what is involved – so that whether one starts on the left or the right is simply something to be remembered – there is considerable risk that they will go wrong. The following example (Farnham-Diggory 1978: 92–3) relates to Ralph, a boy of 11. Although

> he solved mental problems by clever regrouping strategies ...
> Ralph's written computations were seriously in error. He lined up
> numbers from left to right, as in

```
  23
 +5
 ___
  73
```

> He did not know how to carry. For example, given

```
  19
 +16
```

> he began to add from the left, doing $1 + 1 = 2$.
> Next he did $9 + 6 = 15$, which would have given

$$\begin{array}{r} 19 \\ + \ 16 \\ \hline 215 \end{array}$$

but somehow – it is not clear how – he realized that 215 contained too many digits. His solution was simply to ignore the 5! This then gave an answer of 21.

A similar example has been supplied to me by my friend and colleague, Barbara Large.

Joan was a girl of 17. On the Stanford-Binet intelligence test (Terman and Merrill 1960) she had passed four items out of four at 'Average Adult' level, three out of four at 'Superior Adult I' and three out of four at 'Superior Adult II'. She was aiming at going to university. She showed clear indicators of dyslexia on the Bangor Dyslexia Test (Miles 1982), including a failure at 'three digits reversed' ('137' when asked to say '371' backwards). During tuition she was given the following sums: (i) 'Subtract 52 from 103' and (ii) 'Subtract 27 from 36'. Her work was set out as follows:

$$\begin{array}{r} 103 \\ 52 \\ \hline 672 \end{array}$$

and

$$\begin{array}{r} 36 \\ 27 \\ \hline 1? \end{array}$$

It will be seen that in the first sum she has started on the left, subtracted 5 from 11 to get 6, subtracted 2 from 9 to get 7, and subtracted 1 from 3 to get 2. In the second sum this procedure has lead to defeat: she has subtracted 2 from 3 to leave 1 but has realized that 7 cannot be subtracted from 6.

Other examples of directional errors will be found in Miles (1983: 115–16). For instance, that made by a 15-year-old who had said to his parents – in the far off days when petrol was 74p per gallon – 'That petrol's reasonable – forty-seven.' There is also a dramatic report by Street (1976) in which she describes some of the ways in which her uncertainties over left and right contributed in her child-hood to sheer confusion when she was asked to do subtraction sums. There can be little doubt, in general, that the left–right problems which affect dyslexics in other ways also add to the difficulties of calculation.

A final puzzling characteristic of dyslexics requires mention. Spring and Capps (1974: 782) speak of 'the common clinical observation that dyslexic children are specifically impaired on tasks requiring perception of verbal material, while they evidence no dramatic inability to function in an environment of concrete stimuli'. Miles and Ellis (1981) have noted that some dyslexics, when given a task such as 'Touch my right hand with your left hand', sometimes turn in their seats. In the normal way this task requires two separate acts of symbolism – a left–right discrimination in oneself and a left–right discrimination on the person sitting opposite. A person who turns in his seat, however, is thereby reducing one of the acts of symbolism to an act of matching, and this, for a dyslexic, is much easier. In the words of Miles and Ellis (ibid.: 236), 'doing, real or imagined, is a substitute for naming'. In view of this characteristic it seems important that dyslexics should be encouraged to *do* mathematics – that is, operate with concrete objects – rather than try to commit to memory a large number of routines for dealing with symbols. This is a topic to which I shall return in Chapter 6, where I describe some of my experiences when I used structured materials such as Dienes blocks. Dienes himself (1964: 139) has stressed that 'doing' needs to come first. What constitutes bad teaching practice, in his view, is 'the introduction and manipulation of symbolism before adequate experience has been enjoyed of that which is symbolized'. Although he was not talking specifically about the needs of dyslexics, and although starting with 'doing' seems desirable in the case of teaching mathematics to any child, in the case of the dyslexic a failure to do so is likely to be disastrous.

From the evidence cited the following are conclusions which can be accepted with a reasonable degree of confidence:

(i)   All or most dyslexics have mathematical difficulties of some kind, but these can be overcome to varying degrees and in some cases dyslexics can become extremely successful mathematicians.

(ii) They are likely to have problems in their immediate memory for 'number facts', and where it is necessary they may resort to compensatory strategies such as counting on their fingers or putting marks on paper.

(iii) They have difficulty in learning their tables and, in reciting them, may lose the place or become confused.

(iv) They may also lose the place in adding up columns of numbers.

(v) Their difficulties over 'left' and 'right' may affect their calculations.

(vi) They are helped if the basic concepts (addition, and so on) are introduced with concrete examples (adding and taking away blocks, for instance); otherwise the notation is far harder to understand.

It is also likely – though the evidence is not conclusive – that many of them will take longer to learn the meaning of some of the basic symbols, and that even when this knowledge has been acquired they will continue to falter and show uncertainty if the task becomes at all complex. Difficulties over place value, over the zero and over the placing of commas in numbers above 1000 are typical examples (see also Joffe 1983).

THE CONCEPT OF DYSCALCULIA

A widely held view is that there are two separate syndromes, one called 'dyslexia' and one called 'dyscalculia'. It then would be pertinent to ask how many dyslexics are also dyscalculic and how many dyscalculics are (or are not) dyslexic.

To raise the issue in this form, however, is misleading. The central notion of a syndrome is a group of signs, any one of which is insignificant on its own but which, taken in conjunction, form a distinctive pattern. That dyslexia is a syndrome in this sense cannot be doubted. In the case of dyscalculia the matter is far less certain.

Extensive studies of calculation difficulties have been carried out by the Czech neuropsychologist, Ladislav Kosc (see in particular Kosc 1974, and for a detailed description of his work, Sharma and Loveless 1986). The following quotation (Kosc 1974: 165) will serve as a brief summary of his views:

Developmental dyscalculia is a structural disorder of mathematical abilities which has its origin in a genetic or congenital disorder of those parts of the brain that are the direct anatomico-physiological substrate of the maturation of the mathematical abilities adequate to age, without a simultaneous disorder of general mental functions.

It is worth noting that although the word 'dyscalculia', if taken literally, might be expected to mean 'difficulty with calculation', Kosc's account refers to the impairment of *mathematical* skills, and this clearly implies something wider. An important point about mathematics (as opposed simply to calculation), however, is the wide range of different skills that are called for. Thus although it is conceivable that there is a specialized brain centre which underlies these skills and leaves all other skills unaffected, the idea does not seem prima facie likely. It is perhaps rather like looking for a centre which underlies 'memory' simpliciter even though the situations in which we use the word 'remember' are extremely varied.

With regard to *developmental* dyscalculia Kosc writes:

> In principle ... developmental dyscalculia ought to involve only those disorders of mathematical abilities which are the consequence of an impairment (hereditary or congenital) of the growth dynamics of the brain centers which are the organic substrate of mathematical abilities
>
> (Sharma and Loveless 1986: 49)

Now it would be rash to exclude the possibility that there are some children who for organic reasons show a disability which selectively affects their mathematics but none of their other skills. Once again, however, in view of the many different intellectual requirements necessary for mathematics, it is hard to believe that there is no overlap into other areas. Thus if a person starts an addition sum on the left instead of on the right, is it conceivable that his awareness of 'left' and 'right' in non-mathematical contexts will be wholly unaffected? Similarly, if a person 'forgets where he has got to' in adding up a column of digits, is it conceivable that he would never display any comparable evidence of forgetting when asked to memorize a list of words? Yet if one uses a 'syndrome' word such as 'dyscalculia' purely descriptively, this will at best add nothing to the description itself, since 'suffers from dyscalculia' would mean no more than 'is weak at mathematics', while at worst the illusion is created of some 'permanent condition' which is then erroneously postulated as the cause of the difficulties. These arguments also hold in the case of 'dysgraphia'.

Similar objections have, of course, been levelled at the concept of 'dyslexia', namely that it masquerades as an explanation or as a permanent condition when all we know is that the person has difficulty with reading and spelling. There is ample evidence, however, that dyslexia is a genuine syndrome: it has a physical basis and its manifestations are alike in being the consequences of a difficulty at the phonological level (see the first section). In the case of 'dyscalculia' no such evidence has been adduced; and at least as far as the phenomena described in this chapter are concerned the term seems unnecessary.

REFERENCES

Ackerman, P.T., Anhalt, J.M. and Dykman, R.A. (1986) 'Arithmetic automatization failure in children with attention and reading disorders: associations and sequels', *J. Learning Disabilities* 19(4), 222–32.

Ashcraft, M.H. and Fierman, B.A. (1982) 'Mental addition in third, fourth, and sixth graders', *J. Exp. Child Psychol*, 33, 216–34.

Catts, H.W. (1989) 'Phonological processing deficits and reading disabilities', in A.G. Kamhi and H.W. Catts (eds) *Reading Disabilities: A Developmental Language Perspective*, Boston, Little, Brown & Co.

Critchley, M. (1970) *The Dyslexic Child*, London, Heinemann Medical Books.

Critchley, M. and Critchley, E.A. (1978) *Dyslexia Defined*, London, Heinemann Medical Books.

DeFries, J.C., Fulker, D.W. and LaBuda, M.C. (1987) 'Evidence for a genetic aetiology in reading disability twins', *Nature* 329, 537–9.

Dienes, Z.P. (1964) *The Power of Mathematics*, London, Hutchinson Educational.

Done, D.J. and Miles, T.R. (1978) 'Learning, memory, and dyslexia', in M.M. Gruneberg, P.E. Morris and R.N. Sykes (eds) *Practical Aspects of Memory*, London, Academic Press.

Done, D.J. and Miles, T.R. (1988) 'Age of word acquisition in developmental dyslexics as determined by response latencies in a picture naming task', in M.M. Gruneberg, P.E. Morris and R.N. Sykes (eds) *Practical Aspects of Memory: Current Research and Issues* 2, Chichester, Wiley.

Elliott, C.D., Murray, D.J. and Pearson, L.S. (1979) *The British Ability Scales* Windsor, NFER – Nelson.

Ellis, N.C. and Miles, T.R. (1977) 'Dyslexia as a limitation in the ability to process information', *Bulletin of the Orton Society* 27, 72–81.

Ellis, N.C. and Miles, T.R. (1981) 'A lexical encoding deficiency I', in G. Th. Pavlidis and T.R. Miles (eds) *Dyslexia Research and its Applications to Education*, Chichester, Wiley.

Farnham-Diggory, S. (1978) *Learning Disabilities*, London, Fontana Paperbacks.

Finucci, J.M. and Childs, B. (1981) 'Are there really more dyslexic boys than girls?' in A. Ansara, N. Geschwind, A.M. Galaburda, M. Albert and N. Gartrell (eds) *Sex Differences in Dyslexia*, Towson, Orton Dyslexia Society.

Finucci, J.M., Guthrie, J.T., Childs, A.L., Abbey, H. and Childs, B. (1976) 'The genetics of specific reading disability', *Annals of Human Genetics* 40, 1–23.

Fleischner, J.E., Garnett, K. and Shepherd, M.J. (1982) 'Proficiency in arithmetic basic facts computation of learning disabled and nondisabled children', *Focus on Learning Problems in Mathematics* 4(2), 47–56.

Galaburda, A.M. (1989) 'Ordinary and extraordinary brain development: anatomical variation in developmental dyslexia', *Annals of Dyslexia*, 39, 67–80.

Griffiths, J.M. (1980) 'Basic arithmetic processes in the dyslexic child', M. Ed. Dissertation, University of Wales.

Hallgren, B. (1950) 'Specific dyslexia (congenital word blindness). A clinical and genetic study', *Acta Psychiatrica et Neurologica* Supplementum 65, i–xi and 1–287.

Hermann, K. (1959) *Reading Disability,* Copenhagen, Munksgaard.

Hinshelwood, J. (1917) *Congenital Word-Blindness,* London, H.K. Lewis.

Jansons, K.M. (1988) 'A personal view of dyslexia and of thought without language', in L. Weiskrantz (ed.) *Thought Without Language,* Oxford, Oxford University Press.

Joffe, L.S. (1981) 'School mathematics and dyslexia: aspects of the inter-relationship', PhD thesis, University of Aston in Birmingham.

Joffe, L.S. (1983) 'School mathematics and dyslexia – a matter of verbal labelling, generalisation, horses and carts', *Cambridge Journal of Education* 13(3), 22–7.

Joffe, L.S. (1990) 'The mathematical aspects of dyslexia: a recap of general issues and some implications for teaching', *Links* 15(2), 7–10.

Kamhi, A.G. and Catts, H.W. (1989) *Reading Disabilities: A Developmental Language Perspective,* Boston, Little, Brown & Co.

Kosc, L. (1974) 'Developmental dyscalculia', *J. Learning Disabilities,* 7(3), 164–77.

MacMeeken, M. (1939) *Ocular Dominance in Relation to Developmental Aphasia,* London, University of London Press.

Miles, T.R. (1982) *The Bangor Dyslexia Test,* Cambridge, Learning Development Aids.

Miles, T.R. (1983) *Dyslexia: The Pattern of Difficulties,* Oxford, Blackwell.

Miles, T.R. (1987) *Understanding Dyslexia,* Bath, Bath Educational Publishers.

Miles, T.R. and Ellis, N.C. (1981) 'A lexical encoding deficiency II', in G. Th. Pavlidis and T.R. Miles (eds) *Dyslexia Research and its Applications to Education,* Chichester, Wiley.

Miles, T.R. and Miles, E. (1990) *Dyslexia: A Hundred Years On,* Buckingham, Open University Press.

Morgan, W.P. (1896) 'A case of congenital word blindness', *Brit. Med. J.* 2, 1378.

Naidoo, S. (1972) *Specific Dyslexia,* London, Pitman.

Orton, S.T. (1937) *Reading, Writing and Speech Problems in Children,* New York, W.W. Norton.

Pritchard, R.A., Miles, T.R., Chinn, S.J. and Taggart, A.T. (1989) 'Dyslexia and knowledge of number facts', *Links* 14(3), 17–20.

Raven, J.C. (1958) *Standard Progressive Matrices,* London, H.K. Lewis.

Raven, J.C. (1965) *Advanced Progressive Matrices*, London, H.K. Lewis.

Richards, I.L. (1985) 'Dyslexia: a study of developmental and maturational factors associated with a specific cognitive profile', PhD thesis, University of Aston in Birmingham.

Rugel, R.P. (1974) 'WISC sub-test scores of disabled readers', *J. Learning Disabilities*, 7, 48–55.

Sharma, M.C. and Loveless, E.J. (1986) 'The work of Dr Ladislav Kosc on dyscalculia', *Focus on Learning Problems in Mathematics* 8(3, 4), 47–119.

Snowling, M. (1987) *Dyslexia: A Cognitive Developmental Perspective*, Oxford, Blackwell.

Spache, G.D. (1976) *Investigating Issues of Reading Disabilities*, Boston, Allyn & Bacon.

Spring, C. and Capps, C. (1974) 'Encoding speed, rehearsal, and probed recall of dyslexic boys', *J. Educ. Psychol.* 66, 780–6.

Steeves, K.J. (1983) 'Memory as a factor in the computational efficiency of dyslexic children with high abstract reasoning ability', *Annals of Dyslexia* 33, 141–52.

Street, J. (1976) 'Sequencing and directional confusion in arithmetic', *Dyslexia Review* 15, 16–19.

Terman, L.M. and Merrill, M.A. (1960) *Stanford-Binet Intelligence Scale*, London, Harrap.

Thomson, M.E. (1982) 'The assessment of children with specific reading difficulties (dyslexia) using the British Ability Scales', *Brit. J. Psychol.* 73, 461–78.

Thomson, M.E. (1984) *Developmental Dyslexia*, London, Whurr.

Vellutino, F.R. (1979) *Dyslexia: Theory and Research*, Cambridge, Mass., MIT Press.

Vellutino, F.R. (1987) 'Dyslexia', *Scientific American* 256(3), 20–7.

Webster, R.E. (1979) 'Visual and aural short-term memory capacity deficits in mathematics disabled students', *J. Educ. Research* 72(5), 277–83.

Wechsler, D. (1969) *Wechsler Intelligence Scale for Children (WISC-R)*, New York, Psychological Corporation.

NOTES

1. *Annals of Dyslexia* is obtainable from The Orton Dyslexia Society, 724, York Road, Baltimore, Maryland 21204, USA.
2. *Focus on Learning Problems in Mathematics* is obtainable from the Center for the Teaching of Mathematics, PO Box 3149, Framingham, Massachusetts 01701, USA.

Chapter 2

Individual diagnosis and cognitive style

S.J. Chinn

INTRODUCTION: THE USE OF TESTS

Standardized tests can be either norm based or criterion referenced. A norm-based test is one which provides an 'achievement age'; that is to say, it compares the achievement of a particular child on the test with the achievements of his peers. In contrast, a criterion-referenced test is designed to test if set criteria of achievement have been met, for example, the ability to add two three-digit numbers with one 'carrying'.

The information provided by a norm-based test is of value in that it shows how far the child is ahead of or behind his peers in mathematics. In the case of dyslexics, however, scores giving their 'mathematics age' should not be used uncritically, and certainly not in isolation. Additional diagnosis is essential.

In particular it is important to consider the significance not just of the total score but of success or failure at individual items. A norm-based test is in fact standardized by being given to a large sample of children drawn at random from a larger population. If the results do not fit the normal distribution curve the items are changed until they do so. This sometimes results in the inclusion of decidedly 'abnormal' items, some of which may present distinctive problems to the dyslexic. An example of such an item is:

$$10.9 + 9.01 + 19.19$$

One can learn from such an item (which is taken from France 1979) whether the child is able to avoid confusions between different but similar notations; but, as the author would no doubt agree, in view of the many different sub-skills which are involved, it would be absurd to claim that it simply tests 'ability to add' and nothing more.

Similar caution is necessary in the case of the Wide Range Achievement Test (WRAT) (Jastak and Jastak 1978). This is one of the most frequently used tests in the USA. It presents the child with a number of increasingly difficult mathematics problems – the increase in difficulty coming very quickly. There is a tight time limit; the items are presented in very close format, and there is no room to show any steps used in reaching an answer. This type of presentation creates problems for any child, but particularly for the dyslexic who, more than his peers, may be unsure as to the right boundaries between the symbols.

These difficulties can, of course, be avoided if care is taken in interpreting the data. Even then, however, it should be remembered that some dyslexics may 'panic' at the prospect of being tested and that for a variety of reasons their performance may fluctuate on different occasions. It is of importance for teachers to recognize that a test does not always test what it sets out to test. A failure on a mathematics problem may be due to a cause which does not have anything to do with actual mathematical skill.

Criterion-referenced tests do not, as such, emphasize comparison with the performance of the child's peers, though it is, of course, possible to build in 'norm reference' by specifying what an average child is expected to achieve at a given age. In any case there have to be some arbitrary decisions as to which criteria are to be tested. Wilson (1969), for example, broke down the addition of whole numbers into 25 separate sequentially-ordered steps, of which the last six are given here for illustration purposes:

(20) Column of 1 and 2-digit addends, no renaming $(12 + 4 + 3)$
(21) Two 2-place addends, no renaming, 3-place sum $(45 + 83)$
(22) Renaming more than one ten $(49 + 49 + 28 + 28)$
(23) Renaming hundreds $(275 + 152)$
(24) Renaming a ten and a hundred $(399 + 276)$
(25) Renaming thousands $(3,521 + 4,803)$

It is a consequence of this procedure, however, that if one is to obtain an adequate measure of progress the test would have to be impossibly long, since one could scarcely use fewer than two or three items for each criterion and still have confidence in the results.

It is another limitation of criterion-referenced tests that they do not look at the possible existence of error patterns. Borasi (1985) has interestingly suggested that we should consider errors as 'windows' by means of which we can get to know a person's conception of mathematics. The subject of error patterns has also been treated comprehensively by Ashlock (1982). Ashlock points out, in particular, that it is important to examine the child's *wrong* answers, since this is where the teacher can determine if concepts have been misunderstood or algorithms not mastered; and it is then possible to start on the process of correction. There is the further benefit that misconceptions can be stopped before they have become too deeply ingrained. I myself have noted that many schools still use large numbers of problems involving a particular operation; and if a child has adopted an incorrect algorithm, and the teacher does not check the first few examples, there are plenty of opportunities for repeating the error. Here, too, dyslexics, with their poor concentration in class and their less secure knowledge of number facts, are particularly at risk. The following is an example, taken from the France test. The sum was:

$$13.4 + 5$$

In an unpublished survey I myself noted the errors made on this item. The most common one was to rewrite the sum as:

$$\frac{\begin{array}{r} 13.4 \\ +5 \end{array}}{13.9}$$

Cherkes-Julkowski (1985) has suggested that teachers may attribute this kind of error to the learning-disabled child's seemingly rigid or dogmatic thinking, whereas a better explanation may be that he has only a limited number of algorithms at his disposal, some of which he may be able to apply only mechanically, that is, without fully understanding them. If this is so it would account, according to Cherkes-Julkowski, for the high percentage of *systematic* errors made by learning-disabled students.

Also, if an alleged 'test of mathematics' contains a large number of similar items, a little selective tuition on such items would seemingly produce a considerable increase in 'mathematics age'. Clearly such a statistic would be seriously misleading.

In general, if after giving a pupil a test the teacher considers only the score and not the types of error she is losing valuable information. Tests may be failed for many different reasons; and if two pupils both fail a particular item, it by no means follows that they are at the same level of understanding.

It follows from all this that, if the teacher is to be fully aware of the pupil's level of mathematics, a different approach to assessment is needed. In this connection the work of the Arithmetic Clinic, University of Maryland, is particularly impressive and provides many useful ideas (Wilson 1976; Wilson and Sadowski 1976). Full diagnosis requires a closer look at how children (and for that matter adults) *actually do* mathematics − at the errors which they make, and at the background skills which they bring to each problem. This diagnosis takes time, something not always available to teachers; and to allow for individual variation the teacher may need to build on-going diagnosis into the teaching programme. Hence arises the key diagnostic question, 'How did you work it out?' and the recognition that there may be important individual differences in cognitive style.

COGNITIVE STYLE: INCHWORMS AND GRASSHOPPERS

Two American high school teachers (Bath and Knox 1984) had noticed that some of their students (among them dyslexics) responded better to Bath's teaching style and methods while others responded better to Knox's. Analysis of the two teaching styles led to the development of the 'grasshopper' and 'inchworm' theory, which is in effect an account of individual differences in the way in which people do mathematics.

The main characteristics of the two styles are summarized in Table 2.1, taken from the *Test of Cognitive Style in Mathematics* (TCSM) (Bath *et al.* 1986). This is a test in which the subject is given 20 different sorts of mathematical problem and after completion of each is asked, 'How did you do that?' The answer to this question produces the diagnostic information needed to determine cognitive style.

Here are two examples to illustrate the two styles:

Example 1:   A mental arithmetic problem

What is 235 − 97?

The *inchworm* takes the numbers exactly as they are written and looks for a method to fit the problem. In this particular case it is likely that he will visualize the problem as if it were written on paper:

$$
\begin{array}{r}
^{1}2\overset{12}{\cancel{3}}5 \\
-\ 97 \\
\hline
138
\end{array}
$$

The solution is obtained by starting at the units, $5 - 7$, which involves 'renaming' the tens. 35 becomes 25, and the unit subtraction becomes $15 - 7$, which is 8. The tens column is now $2 - 9$, which also requires 'renaming': the 2 becomes 12, and $12 - 9 = 3$.

Table 2.1 Cognitive styles of the inchworm and the grasshopper

	Inchworm	Grasshopper
I. Analysing and identifying the problem	1. Focuses on parts, attends to detail and separates. 2. Objective of looking at facts to determine useful formula.	1. Holistic, forms concepts and puts together. 2. Objective of looking at facts to determine an estimate of answer or range of restrictions.
II. Methods of solving the problem	3. Formula, recipe oriented. 4. Constrained focusing using a single method or serial-ordered steps along one route (Rifle approach), generally in one direction – forward. 5. Uses numbers exactly as given. 6. Tending to add and multiply: resists subtraction and division. 7. Tending to use paper and pencil to compute.	3. Controlled exploration. 4. Flexible focusing using multi-methods or paths, frequently occurring simultaneously (Shot gun), generally reversing or working back from an answer and trying new routes. 5. Adjusts, breaks down/ builds up numbers to make an easier calculation. 6. Tending to subtract. 7. Tending to perform all computation mentally.
III. Verification	8. Verification unlikely; if done, uses same procedure or method.	8. Likely to verify; probably uses alternate procedure or method.

Source: Bath *et al.* 1986.

The hundreds column has become 1, which means that the final answer is 138.

This style is method-orientated. The user must bring to the problem a good working memory and a good knowledge of basic number facts; in the absence of this knowledge the load on working memory is very heavy. The actual algorithm used will usually depend on what has been taught. Thirty years ago the most likely method to be used would have been that of 'equal additions' where the working would be set out as follows:

$$2\,3\,\overset{\scriptscriptstyle '}{5}$$
$$\underset{\scriptscriptstyle 1}{-}\,\overset{\scriptscriptstyle \circ}{9}\,7$$
$$\overline{1\,3\,8}$$

More recently schools have used Dienes blocks as a concrete aid, in which case 'renaming' will predominate as the method used.

In contrast the *grasshopper* method would be as follows:

(i)   97 is rounded up to 100
(ii)   235 − 100 = 135
(iii) 135 + 3 = 138 (with the 3 adjusting the 100 back to 97)

This style is answer-orientated. The numbers are adjusted to suit the style and reduce the load on the working memory. Those who work in this way often find it difficult to show their method in writing, and in some cases an unsympathetic teacher may mark them down for this.

Example 2:   A geometric/visual problem

What is the area of the shaded part of Figure 2.1?

Inchworm method   A subject who brings to the problem a knowledge of triangles, squares, and their areas is likely to see the 'dog' as a triangle, a square, and two rectangles. The 'dog' is seen as made up of parts, and the initial approach is to identify formulae. Again it is what the subject knows as well as his style that controls the method used to solve the problem. These two factors are inter-woven.

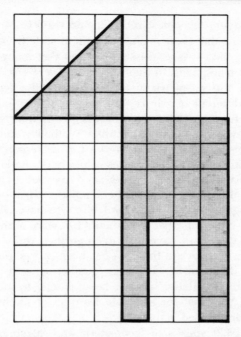

Figure 2.1 The dog problem: what is the area of the shaded part of the figure?

According to formula:

area of triangle: $\frac{1}{2} \times 4 \times 4 = 8$
area of square: $4 \times 4 = 16$
area of rectangles: $2 \times (4 \times 1) = 8$

Total   32

It should be noted that the order of adding is likely to be sequential and not adjusted to make the numbers easier to add (as might be done, for instance, if the pupil used number bonds which add up to 10, viz. $16 + 4 = 20$, $20 + 8 + 4 = 32$).

Grasshopper method   A child less comfortable with formulae and number operations may seek some way to redesign and simplify the problem. Thus the triangle is half of a 4×4 square, as also is the gap in between the two 'legs'. The figure is then transformed into an 8×4 rectangle.

After studying test-retest reliability on the TCSM, the authors have suggested that there is a continuum of style from the extreme inchworm to the extreme grasshopper and that many children are consistent in using a mix of the two (Bath *et al.* 1986). I myself have noticed that the geometric/visual section of the test frequently produces a different bias in cognitive style; and it is possible that these items require relatively less access to number skills and are testing ability to visualize rather than symbolic representation of numbers. This, however, is a matter for further research.

I have also noticed, from studies of teachers' marking of typical grasshopper and inchworm answers, and from reactions to my own lectures on this topic, that teachers no less than pupils have a preferred cognitive style; and if this is not to have adverse consequences it is important that they should be aware of the fact.

Other investigators have also distinguished different cognitive styles. The major work in this area has been carried out by Sharma (1989) who distinguishes between 'qualitative' and 'quantitative' thinkers (the 'quantitative' thinker being similar to the inchworm). Sharma suggests that for adequate learning of mathematics both approaches are needed.

Harvey (1982) speaks of 'geometers' and 'algebraists', thereby hinting at potential areas of strength and weakness. Polya (1962) suggests four styles: 'groping', 'bright idea', 'algebra', and 'generalization', though it would not be unreasonable to combine them in pairs, 'groping' and 'bright idea' being equivalent to grasshopper style, and 'algebra' and 'generalization' being equivalent to inchworm style. In that case his conclusions are in line with those of Bath *et al.*, Sharma and Harvey.

It has also been hypothesized that cognitive style may be related to hemispheric specialization. The suggestion is that the right brain controls holistic, grasshopper thinking, and that the left brain is responsible for inchworm, logical, sequential thinking (see, for instance, Wheatley *et al.* 1978, Grow and Johnson 1983).

Several writers, notably Krutetskii (1976), have emphasized the need for flexibility in tackling mathematical problems. Similarly Kubrick and Rudnick (1980) state that teachers should allow for and encourage a wide variety of approaches, ideas, questions, solutions and discussions.

There are also interesting analogies with the ideas of de Bono, who speaks of 'lateral' and 'vertical' styles of thinking. The following passage is worth quoting in full:

Lateral thinking is quite distinct from vertical thinking, which is the traditional type of thinking. In vertical thinking one moves forward by sequential steps, each of which must be justified. . . . In lateral thinking one may have to be wrong at some stage in order to obtain a correct solution. Lateral thinking does not exclude other pathways. Both types of thinking are required. They are complementary.

(de Bono 1970: 41)

CONSEQUENCES FOR PUPILS

Earlier in the chapter it was suggested that the way in which a problem is solved depends in part on what the pupil has brought to the situation, in particular what algorithms he has available and what is his knowledge of basic number facts. The ways in which these factors interact with cognitive style is of importance for the teaching of mathematics to any pupil and to dyslexics in particular.

Other relevant factors are: strength or weakness of short-term memory, reading skill, willingness to write down on paper and ease and facility in doing so, ability to use a variety of strategies, and a general facility with numbers.

A grasshopper who has few basic facts available at instant recall is likely to have developed strategies which compensate for this. Indeed, the interaction of style and strategy is one of mutual support. His explanations, if he provides them, are less sequentially logical and often more difficult to articulate than more formula-based methods. He is likely to be good at estimating and less good at answering blocks of questions on the same topic. As has been indicated, he is very answer-orientated.

An inchworm with good basic fact knowledge is unlikely to be an inspired problem solver, but will probably have few difficulties in surviving in mathematics. As has been indicated, he is very process/formula orientated.

The pupil most at risk is the dyslexic inchworm, that is, the inchworm with poor basic fact knowledge and poor short-term memory and long-term retrieval problems. If the rote learning of number facts is difficult, the obvious alternative is to devise strategies. The idea of strategies, however, belongs more to grasshopper than to inchworm style, and the teaching of them to an inchworm may not be easy. Alternatively, if one gets the pupil to proceed – inchworm-like – through successive stages (as is done, for instance when

Wilson, 1969, categorizes whole number addition into 25 progressive steps, see above), the cost in terms of time and effort is likely to be considerable, and in any case this procedure will not develop number facility or estimating skills.

THE CONSEQUENCES FOR TEACHERS

Both for teachers and for learners there are potential problems in having an 'extreme' style, whether inchworm or grasshopper. Bath and Knox (personal communication) both had to modify their teaching styles or at least work together with students (team-teach) so as to avoid over-emphasis on one style.

Lankford (1974) has expressed concern that 'unorthodox' methods used by children may be discouraged, while Hart (1978) has noted that pupils may not naturally use the methods which their teachers demonstrate. Awareness on the part of the teacher that there are variations in individual style is essential.

More recently Hart (1989) has examined children's ability to understand the concepts or rules being demonstrated and developed. The results are to be published in book form. Hart has suggested that a suitable subtitle for the book might be *Sums are Sums and Bricks are Bricks*. This subtitle implies that children do not necessarily make connections between concrete manipulatives and abstract numbers. Thus the step-by-step logic of a teacher's lesson may be lost on her grasshopper student, while the global overview and conceptual discourse of another teacher may be lost on an inchworm student. The development of a concept may be more effective if use is made of a grasshopper overview, followed by an inchworm detailed examination, followed by a grasshopper review. Both styles should be addressed together during the lesson.

Sharma (personal communication) has suggested that pupils with predominantly inchworm characteristics far outnumber those with grasshopper characteristics. It seems reasonable to suppose that dyslexics, because of their memory limitations and problems of symbolic representation, would on the whole tend to be grasshoppers; and if this is so they would be seriously at risk in a group where the teacher and most of the pupils were inchworms.

It is an obvious requirement that the teaching of mathematics to dyslexics should be multisensory (Steeves 1979). In addition, however, this teaching has to be applicable to a continuum of learning styles; and the differences in style need to be explicitly acknowledged by the teacher. Inchworms need to learn grasshopper skills and strategies, while grasshoppers need to learn how to handle standard algorithms, classify problems into similar groups, and document their methods if they are to become more successful at school mathematics.

TEACHING TO BOTH COGNITIVE STYLES

To illustrate how one can teach to both styles I have chosen two examples. The first relates to the teaching of times tables, while the second – which at first glance may seem an unpromising topic – is concerned with the inter-conversion of metric and British units of measurement.

Teaching times table facts

An inchworm is likely to favour learning the times tables by rote. For a dyslexic this would normally require a multisensory approach: thus he would say the fact aloud (for example, 'two fours are eight'), write down the figures ('2 × 4 = 8'), and read what he has written. The spoken, heard, visual, and motor inputs to the brain would all come into play.

The ARROW technique (Lane and Chinn 1986) is also multi-sensory, but uses a tape recorder and headphones. This technique is an extension of the self-voice echo (Keeney *et al.* 1967).

Often an inchworm can recall a fact only by reciting the whole sequence up to that fact; thus the correct answer to '9 × 2' may be possible for him only after '1 × 2' to '8 × 2' have been chanted. A disadvantage of this method is that it does nothing to promote awareness of the interrelationships between number facts; for example '6 × 2' will not be seen as one more 2 than '5 × 2' (the answer to which is at the end of your arms). The situation is made worse if the child is encouraged to think of the tables as 'the fives', 'the twos', and so on, as though they were isolated chunks of infor-mation. In general this method is inefficient and slow and does not develop any 'feel' for the ways in which numbers behave or any facility in operating with numbers. For a dyslexic in particular it can therefore be very frustrating.

A grasshopper is likely to use a variety of strategies, including some of those described by Ashcroft and myself in Chapter 7 of this book. There may well be a lack of consistency, however, and some of his strategies may be the result of somewhat unsystematic indi-

vidual observations of connections between number facts. Thus the
5 × table may be seen as half the 10 × table (Pritchard *et al.* 1989),
and 6 × 6 may be seen as one six more than 5 × 6 but other
relationships may not be noticed.

Ultimately the teaching of the times tables can be an exercise in
developing both cognitive styles and can thus promote a more
flexible approach to this particular task. The method given below
reinforces the work on block patterns described by Ashcroft and
myself in Chapter 7. Obviously limitations of space and the
reader's tolerance restrict the extent of this description, but I hope
the information given will demonstrate the essentials of what is
involved in teaching to both kinds of cognitive style.

The times table facts are learned from a table square (Figure 2.2).

×	0	1	2	3	4	5	6	7	8	9	10
0	0	0	0	0	0	0	0	0	0	0	0
1	0	1	2	3	4	5	6	7	8	9	10
2	0	2	4	6	8	10	12	14	16	18	20
3	0	3	6	9	12	15	18	21	24	27	30
4	0	4	8	12	16	20	24	28	32	36	40
5	0	5	10	15	20	25	30	35	40	45	50
6	0	6	12	18	24	30	36	42	48	54	60
7	0	7	14	21	28	35	42	49	56	63	70
8	0	8	16	24	32	40	48	56	64	72	80
9	0	9	18	27	36	45	54	63	72	81	90
10	0	10	20	30	40	50	60	70	80	90	100

Figure 2.2 The table square

Notes

1. The square can be given to each pupil as something to which he
   can refer; and he need not be put under pressure to *learn* any of
   the tables. It can be pasted in the back of his exercise book and
   he can be allowed free access to it. The idea is that it takes some
   effort to refer to it but that the effort is immediately rewarded by
   'success', although there is, of course, no special opportunity to
   develop number sense.

2. The table includes the 0 and 1 facts. These are important in their own right and in any case have value later in other areas of mathematics. At no stage should the integrity of mathematics be compromised.
3. The square stops at 100, the 10× table. Eleven, twelve and beyond are calculated by strategies, developed while the pupil is learning the square.

There are 121 facts to learn. One of the principles is to reduce the task to manageable proportions. The 'easy' facts are learned first, namely the 0× and 1× tables.

This gives a first introduction to the commutative property, for example that $3 \times 1 = 1 \times 3$ or that $0 \times 5 = 5 \times 0$. As in the case of all lessons with dyslexics, the teacher should introduce alternative expressions, for instance, 'three times', 'three lots of', 'multiply', 'how many threes in ...?', and so on. These incidentals are important as they act as constant reminders of the language of mathematics and they contribute to the understanding of new concepts.

There is a range of concrete teaching materials available which may be of help (Dienes blocks, Cuisenaire rods, money, and so on). It is important, however, to bear in mind the warning given by Hart (1989) (see above) that the pupil must make the link between the concrete objects and the number symbol. Thus each lesson should use both actual materials and the digits which they represent.

Mastery of the 1× and 0× facts reduces the number of items to be learned from 121 to 81. The table square may be shaded in accordingly.

The ten-times facts may now be introduced. The concept of 'ten' is important (compare Cobb and Wheatley 1988). There are patterns to help – a visual pattern and, with a little licence (for example, 'five' and 'fifty'), an aural pattern. There is a range of trading activities which can be used (trading 10p coins and 1p coins, and so on).

The inchworm will probably focus on the 1:10, 2:20, 3:30 relationship as a series of individual facts. He may need some help to see that the pattern repeats constantly and that he can enter it at any point rather than starting at 1×10 and working up each time.

The grasshopper will normally be comfortable with the pattern of the 10× table, but even so it may be of help to draw his attention to it. Once again one is helping him to be aware of the value of patterns in mathematics.

There are other activities which a creative teacher can use, but this would take us outside the scope of the present chapter.

The task is now down to 64 facts. The commutative property can be mentioned again, and it can be pointed out that this property gives two facts for the price of one!

It is important for developing facility with number that the relationships between numbers are explored and developed. Inchworms tend to accept numbers exactly as they are – that is, as isolated chunks of information, independent of other facts around them. Thus 5 is seen as 5, not half of 10, as a tenth of 50, or as ten times one half. Nor is 15 seen as 10 plus half of 10.

The five-times facts can be taught as half of the ten-times facts, with the additional check of 5 − 0 endings relating to odd and even multipliers.

The two-times facts, which are often learned most easily, can be explored for patterns and relationships to reinforce the learning and further develop number facility. For example the concepts of 'even' and 'odd' numbers can be taught. Also the idea of a reference point mid-way can be introduced to help the inchworm to avoid going back to 1×2 each time. The answer to 5×2 is 10; 5 fingers, 2 hands. Then 6×2 is one more two than ten. The idea that adding and multiplying are linked is also introduced. The repetitive pattern of 2, 4, 6, 8, 0 can be emphasized as the endings for all even numbers.

The link between 5×2 and 6×2 is important. It introduces the child to the idea that numbers can be broken down and adjusted to help with calculations. For the inchworm, therefore, a grasshopper skill is introduced, while for the grasshopper there is the opportunity for learning to rationalize and unify his strategies, since he is explicitly being encouraged to use generalizations and formulae.

Successful learning of strategies for $0\times$, $1\times$, $2\times$, $5\times$, and $10\times$ has reduced the task to the learning of 36 facts. If the nine-times is taught through patterns and by estimating 9 as 10 the figure is reduced to 25. The commutative property (less the squares for 3, 4, 6, 7, and 8) brings the number down to 10.

This method takes a task which is impossible for most dyslexics and reduces it to a reachable goal. In doing so it teaches the inter-relationships of numbers and starts to build an understanding of how they work.

Teaching conversion of units

Both metric and British units are still in common use. A knowledge of the relative values of the two is useful in practice; and there is the opportunity – despite the seemingly unpromising nature of the topic – for teaching several different points, including flexibility in particular (Table 2.2).

The following lessons, among others, can be taught from this chart:

1. The pupil can be made aware of left/right directionality, since he has to move either leftwards or rightwards from the central bold numbers to the correct column.
2. There is the chance to study place values, tens, units and decimals.
3. There is the opportunity to evaluate the precision of all conversions and to consider the need for different levels of accuracy in different circumstances.
4. The issue of comparative values can be raised – 'Which unit gives more?', and 'Which conversion leads to a bigger number, which to a smaller?'
5. There can be discussion of estimations, for example 2 lb for 1 kg.
6. There is the issue of refining estimates. For example, in converting kilograms to pounds a rough estimate is to double the number (see (5), above). The refining involves adding one tenth of the doubled number. This also teaches that 0.2 is one tenth of 2, which is another example of the building up of number concepts.
7. It is possible to teach reference values which are not based on one, for example the awareness that 5 miles approximates to 8 kilometres. From this the lesson can be extended to proportion and algorithms for proportion.
8. Realistic tolerances can be discussed, for example, whether timber measuring 50 mm × 100 mm is acceptable if the specification is 2 inch by 4 inch.
9. There can be discussion of how units are 'extended'; for example distance on its own can be extended to distance ÷ time, that is, speed.

These examples give some ideas for introducing flexibility of topic and style into a lesson. The learner is meeting algorithms, estimates, precise numbers, strategies, evaluation, and techniques of

Table 2.2 Metric conversion tables

The bold figures in the central columns can be read as either the metric or the British measure. Thus 1 inch – 25.4 millimetres; or 1 millimetre – 0.039 inches.

Inches	Millimetres		Yards	Metres		Sq yards	Sq metres		Ounces	Grams		Pints	Litres
0.039	25.4	**1**	1.094	0.914	**1**	1.196	0.836	**1**	0.035	28.350	**1**	1.760	0.568
0.079	50.8	**2**	2.187	1.829	**2**	2.392	1.672	**2**	0.071	56.699	**2**	3.520	1.137
0.118	76.2	**3**	3.281	2.743	**3**	3.588	2.508	**3**	0.106	85.048	**3**	5.279	1.705
0.157	101.6	**4**	4.374	3.658	**4**	4.784	3.345	**4**	0.141	113.398	**4**	7.039	2.273
0.197	127.0	**5**	5.468	4.572	**5**	5.980	4.181	**5**	0.176	141.748	**5**	8.799	2.841
0.236	152.4	**6**	6.562	5.486	**6**	7.176	5.017	**6**	0.212	170.097	**6**	10.559	3.410
0.276	177.8	**7**	7.655	6.401	**7**	8.372	5.853	**7**	0.247	198.446	**7**	12.318	3.978
0.315	203.2	**8**	8.749	7.315	**8**	9.568	6.689	**8**	0.282	226.796	**8**	14.078	4.546
0.354	228.6	**9**	9.843	8.230	**9**	10.761	7.525	**9**	0.317	255.146	**9**	15.838	5.114

Feet	Metres		Miles	Kilometres		Cu feet	Cu metres		Pounds	Kilograms		Gallons	Litres
3.281	0.305	**1**	0.621	1.609	**1**	35.315	0.028	**1**	2.205	0.454	**1**	0.220	4.516
6.562	0.610	**2**	1.243	3.219	**2**	70.629	0.057	**2**	4.409	0.907	**2**	0.440	9.092
9.843	0.914	**3**	1.864	4.828	**3**	105.941	0.085	**3**	6.614	1.361	**3**	0.660	13.638
13.123	1.219	**4**	2.485	6.437	**4**	141.259	0.113	**4**	8.818	1.814	**4**	0.880	18.181
16.404	1.524	**5**	3.107	8.047	**5**	176.573	0.142	**5**	11.023	2.268	**5**	1.100	22.730
19.685	1.829	**6**	3.728	9.656	**6**	211.888	0.170	**6**	13.228	2.722	**6**	1.320	27.277
22.966	2.134	**7**	4.350	11.265	**7**	247.203	0.198	**7**	15.432	3.175	**7**	1.540	31.823
26.247	2.438	**8**	4.971	12.875	**8**	282.517	0.227	**8**	17.637	3.629	**8**	1.760	36.369
29.528	2.743	**9**	5.592	14.484	**9**	317.832	0.255	**9**	19.812	4.082	**9**	1.980	40.915

Conversion factors

To convert to metric, multiply by the factor shown. To convert from metric, divide by the factor. Factors have been rounded for convenience.

Length	
miles: kilometres	1.6093
yards: metres	0.9144
feet: metres	0.3048
inches: millimetres	25.4
inches: centimetres	2.54

Volume	
cubic yards: cubic metres	0.7646
cubic feet: cubic metres	0.0283
cubic inches:	
cubic centimetres	16.3871

Velocity	
miles per hour:	
kilometres per hour	1.6093

Area	
square miles: square kilometres	2.59
square miles: hectares	258.999
acres: square metres	4046.86
acres: hectares	0.4047
square yards: square metres	0.8361
square feet: square metres	0.0929
square feet: square centimetres	929.03
square inches:	
square millimetres	615.16

Fuel consumption	
gallons per mile:	
litres per kilometre	2.825
miles per gallon:	
kilometres per litre	0.354

Mass	
tons: kilograms	1016.05
tons: tonnes	1.0160
hundredweights:	
kilograms	50.8023
pounds: kilograms	0.4536
ounces: grams	28.3495

Capacity	
gallons:	
cubic decimetres	4.5461
gallons: litres	4.546
US barrels: cubic metres	
(for petroleum)	0.159
pints: cubic decimetres	0.5683
pints: litres	0.568

overviewing and checking answers. To dyslexic pupils in particular such things may well provide an exciting challenge.

CONCLUSION

The concept of different learning styles, though relevant in the case of all pupils, is particularly relevant to the teaching of dyslexics. The diagnosis and subsequent remedial programme offered, and even the subsequent mainstream programme, should acknowledge that not all children process numbers in the same way and that children have different batteries of skills and knowledge. The typical dyslexic problems of difficulty in rote learning, short-term memory deficits, and weakness at arranging symbolic material in sequence are likely to make many standard methods and basic facts difficult to learn.

The dyslexic in this position will either start to develop his own strategies, which may not be systematic, efficient or organized, or he may decide to 'give up' on mathematics altogether. The advantage of the inchworm/grasshopper concept is that if it is introduced all pupils will benefit from a greater flexibility in using numbers. They will have a better chance of experiencing success and a wider set of learning experiences from which to develop concepts. The thought of classes divided up into inchworms, grasshoppers, and 'intermediates' (or 'inchhoppers'), is a little bizarre. Instead a flexible programme can be devised which is suitable for both learning styles and appropriate for a wide range of children. Such a programme is likely to be of help not only to dyslexics but to other students also.

REFERENCES

Ashlock, R.B. (1982) *Error Patterns in Computation*, Columbus, Ohio, Merrill.

Bath, J., Chinn, S.J. and Knox, D. (1986) *The Test of Cognitive Style in Mathematics*, New York, Slosson.

Bath, J. and Knox, D. (1984) 'Two styles of performing mathematics', in J. Bath, S.J. Chinn and D. Knox (eds) *Dyslexia: Research and its Applications to the Adolescent*, Bath, Better Books.

Borasi, R. (1985) 'Using errors as springboards for the learning of mathematitics: an introduction', *Focus on Learning Problems in Mathematics* 7(34), 1–15.

Cherkes-Julkowski, M. (1985) 'Metacognitive considerations in mathematics instruction for the learning disabled', in J.F. Cawley (ed.) *Cognitive Strategies and Mathematics for the Learning Disabled*, Rockville, M, Aspen.

Cobb, P. and Wheatley, G. (1988) 'Children's initial understandings of ten',

Focus on Learning Problems in Mathematics 10(3), 1–28.

de Bono, E. (1970) *Lateral Thinking: A Textbook of Creativity*, London, Ward Lock Educational.

France, N. (1979) *Profile of Mathematical Skills*, Windsor, NFER – Nelson.

Grow, M. and Johnson, N. (1983) 'Math learning: the two hemispheres', *Humanistic Education and Development* 22, 30–9.

Hart, K. (1981) *Children's Understanding of Mathematics: 11–16*, London, John Murray.

Hart, K. (1989) 'There is little connection', In P. Ernest (ed.) *Mathematics Teaching: The State of the Art*, Lewes, Falmer Press.

Harvey, R. (1982) *Language Teaching and Learning, No. 6*, Mathematics, London, Ward Lock Educational.

Jastak, J.F. and Jastak, S. (1978) *Wide Range Achievement Test* (revised edn), Wilmington, DE, Jastak Associates.

Keeney, T.J., Cannizzo, S.R. and Flavell, J.H. (1967) 'Spontaneous and induced verbal rehearsal in the recall task', *Child Development* 38(4), 952.

Krutetskii, V.A. (1976) *The Psychology of Mathematical Abilities in Schoolchildren*, Chicago, University of Chicago Press.

Kubrick, S. and Rudnick, J.A. (1980) *Problem Solving – A Handbook for Teachers*, Needham Heights, USA, Allyn & Bacon.

Lane, C. and Chinn, S.J. (1986) 'Learning by self-voice echo', *Academic Therapy* 21(4), 477–81.

Lankford, F.G. (1974) 'What can a teacher learn about a pupil's thinking through oral interviews?' *The Arithmetic Teacher* 22, 26–32.

Polya, G. (1962) *Mathematical Discovery*, New York, Wiley.

Pritchard, R.A., Miles, T.R., Chinn, S.J. and Taggart, A.T. (1989) 'Dyslexia and knowledge of number facts, *Links* 14(3), 17–20.

Sharma, M. (1989) 'Mathematics learning personality', *Math Notebook* 7 (1, 2), 1–10.

Steeves, J. (1979) 'Multi-sensory math: an instructional approach to help the LD child', *Focus on Learning Problems in Mathematics* 1(2), 51–62.

Wheatley, G., Frankland, R., Mitchell, R. and Kraft, R. (1978) 'Hemispheric specialisation and cognitive development: implications for mathematics education', *Journal for Research in Mathematics Education*, 9, 20–32.

Wilson, J. (1969) *Some Guides for Elementary School Mathematics*, Maryland, private publication.

Wilson, J. (1976) *Diagnosis and Treatment in Arithmetic: Beliefs, Guiding Models and Procedures*, Maryland, University of Maryland.

Wilson, J. and Sadowski, B. (1976) (eds) *The Maryland Diagnostic Arithmetic Test and Interview Protocols*, Maryland, University of Maryland.

Chapter 3

Linking language to action

Mary Kibel

A LESSON WITH ALEX

Some years ago, I took a course on teaching mathematics. It was called 'Developing Mathematical Thinking'. As part of the course we had to try various activities with a child and notice his approach. I worked with a dyslexic 14-year-old called Alex. One of the activities was a game called 'Shrink-A-Square'. It had been designed to teach decomposition – the 'borrowing' procedure in subtraction. This game had a surprising effect on Alex. I shall describe it in detail.

We played with Dienes blocks[1] on boards marked in columns with 'hundreds', 'tens' and 'units'. We each started off with a block of 100 which we placed in the hundreds-position on our boards. This was the square that we had to 'shrink'. Then we threw a dice in turn and took away the number we threw. If the subtraction involved decomposition, we had to exchange one large block for ten smaller ones before we could take away. The winner was the first person to end up with no blocks at all.

This was simple enough – but the manipulation of the blocks had to be accompanied by a verbal description of what was happening. If the subtraction involved exchange, we had to accompany the operation with a precise mathematical statement to describe what we were doing – 'I take one ten from the tens-position and exchange it for ten units. I put the ten units in the units-position, and then I take away the six.' The aim of the activity was to encourage children to practise and perfect the language of exchange.

Alex and I took a long time working our way down from 100. It became much too easy, and so to make the game more fun we began closing our eyes as we manipulated the blocks and described what we were doing. Next, we tried describing the whole process, eyes shut, without touching the blocks at all. This proved surprisingly hard for Alex. The temptation to open his eyes and handle the blocks was very strong. He could not sustain the language on its own. But eventually, given time and practice, the verbal explanation became surprisingly easy and the blocks almost superfluous. At this point we transferred to the formal written algorithm. The transition was swift and trouble-free. Alex left that afternoon feeling that we had had an amusing time, nothing more.

But the effect was dramatic. Alex was 14. He had never understood how to do subtraction when this involved 'borrowing'. He regularly took the lowest numbers from the highest, regardless of whether they were on the top or bottom line – and he regularly got his answers wrong! Some time later, he called round and proudly announced, 'I can do those take-aways. They're easy. We've been doing them at school this week and I got the whole lot right. No problem! They're *ace*, they are.'

I was surprised. I gave him a few to do, and sure enough, he worked his way through them faultlessly with great ease and enjoyment. A month later he could still do them and to my knowledge he has not forgotten to this day.

SOME GUIDING PRINCIPLES

I was puzzled by what had happened. Nine years of careful schooling had not taught Alex how to subtract when this involved exchange, and yet the half-hour spent on this simple game had succeeded in getting the concept across in a secure and permanent way. What did the 'Shrink-A-Square' game offer that normal teaching lacked?

Alex was dyslexic – it was possible that certain aspects of the game were particularly relevant to dyslexia and that this was the reason for its success. I felt that this was worth pursuing and analysed the activity more carefully.

One striking feature was that at no point did I have to *tell* Alex what to do. As he worked with the blocks, the procedure for decomposition was obvious and so no verbal explanation was necessary.

Dyslexics have difficulty with language. If mathematics is taught through the medium of language, if children are told what to do and expected to remember a sequence of verbal instructions, then dyslexic children are going to find this hard. We are asking them to rely on an area in which we know they are cognitively weak.

When we translate the procedure into a visual form that can be manipulated and solved spatially, there is an important change of emphasis. We engage non-verbal routes to understanding and reduce the role of language. For a dyslexic, this change of approach could be a particularly helpful one.

Yet the 'Shrink-A-Square' game did not reduce the role of language completely. Rather the reverse – the language and manipulating seemed to work together in a mutually supportive way. Each time Alex went through the procedure for decomposition, he had to describe what he was doing in words. The language reinforced the sequence of actions. This is verbal labelling. It is a strategy that most people use to help them remember things.

We know that dyslexics are poor at verbal labelling. When Alex played the 'Shrink-A-Square' game, he was forced to use this strategy in a very precise and deliberate way. The effect of this could have been to strengthen an area in which he is naturally weak – and this may have helped him remember the sequence of operations needed for the complicated 'borrowing' procedure.

Moreover, there was considerable overlearning of the language. During our half-hour session we played several games and Alex must have repeated the language of exchange some 20 to 30 times! But what is more interesting – the talking ran alongside the manipulating. We were 'tying' the language to visual and kinesthetic images. Alex talked as he handled as he looked. It was multisensory learning.

Dyslexics have difficulty with mathematical terms. The words do not hold meaning easily. For Alex the terms 'exchange', 'tens-position', 'one ten for ten units' became bound to the action. Later, if meaning fades, the words themselves should conjure up clear kinesthetic and visual images of what we were doing. This means that, as well as practising the mathematical language, we were giving it meaning and solidity. We were helping to make it permanent. And we did so in a multisensory way.

These ideas have now become the basis for all the work I do. When I teach mathematics, I try to structure each learning situation in a very deliberate way.

If I teach something new, I never ask children to rely on a sequence of verbal instructions – I never *tell* them what to do. Instead I create a physical representation of the concept and give them problems to solve by manipulation. This increases opportunities for non-verbal learning and reduces dependence on language.

I strengthen the role of verbal labelling by arranging for language to run alongside the manipulating. I try to make this a prominent and challenging part of the activity by insisting that the language is precise and allowing no short cuts!

Strong kinesthetic and visual images should underlie mathematical terms. I always arrange for considerable overlearning of the language, and ensure that abstract terms are linked to a concrete base.

None of this is new, of course. Teachers have always maintained that children learn best by doing, particularly in the early years. The main thrust of the course 'Developing Mathematical Thinking'[2] was precisely this. Concepts should not be passed on ready-made. They should be allowed to grow in concrete situations and only later should formal written work take place.

What I have tried to show is that this approach has very clear advantages for dyslexics. It gives solid support in areas where language is weak. For children like Alex who repeatedly forget despite years of careful teaching this may be a safer way in which to learn.

ALLOWING TIME FOR CONCEPTS TO FORM

In a moment I shall give examples of how these ideas work out in practice, but before I do so, I would like to look more closely at an important aspect of the 'Shrink-A-Square' game – the concrete nature of the learning and the length of time that it took.

Alex and I spent a full half-hour on the 'Shrink-A-Square' game and during that time the learning passed through several interesting stages.

At first the language itself was difficult – the words were unfamiliar, and the length and precision of the statement awkward to cope with. As fluency developed, Alex began to talk his way through the procedure with confidence. Yet for a long time the language remained curiously dependent on the action. He could not hold the idea in his head. When he tried to describe the process with his eyes closed, he faltered and the description became muddled and confused. The need to handle the blocks and look at the visual layout was very great indeed. Alex seemed to understand quite clearly what he was doing, but the understanding was embedded[3] in the concrete situation. The concept could not stand alone.

Eventually, of course, the need for tangible support did fall away. Handling the blocks became unnecessary and almost annoying. Alex could explain the whole procedure, eyes shut, with no difficulty at all. This was the point at which he mastered the process. An internal model had formed. The 'Shrink-A-Square' game had done its work.

It was then that we changed to normal written subtraction. Alex found this easy to do. Even an unexpected nought on the top line presented no problem. Alex could 'see' that one hundred needed to be exchanged for 10 tens. He could dip down into more concrete levels of thinking. His newly-won concept was functioning well. It had evolved slowly in a concrete situation and was very solidly underpinned. But it had taken a surprisingly long time.

Perhaps the most helpful thing about the 'Shrink-A-Square' game was that, by chance, it held Alex in a concrete learning situation for an unusual length of time. It was long enough for the whole process of concept formation to be fully complete by the time he came to tackle formal subtraction. The result of this was that Alex did not have to remember a set of rules, and when he met an unexpected problem – the nought on the top line – he did not need to ask me what to do. He was able to work things out for himself by drawing on his sound underlying knowledge of the full procedure for subtraction.

Perhaps the reason for his sudden competence was that he no longer needed to remember a sequence of verbal instructions. He could work directly from a basic understanding of the process, and when the need arose he was able to translate back to more concrete ways of thinking.

Many dyslexic youngsters do become quite good at mathematics. They too seem to work in this way, often solving problems by unconventional methods because they prefer to work from the underlying concept, the *sense* in the situation, rather than by following the teacher's rule. Perhaps these children have discovered for themselves that they can avoid their linguistic limitation by working in more direct and concrete ways.

Another factor may be involved here. It is possible that, because of a generalized weakness in language, dyslexics have difficulty with the process of concept formation itself. Their thinking may remain embedded in concrete situations for longer than is usual with other children. The jump from concrete to abstract may happen less easily for them. In the 'Shrink-A-Square' game, Alex spent a very long time at the manipulating stage of the learning. It was far longer than I would have thought necessary. Yet this may have provided him, by chance, with just the opportunity he needed.

So my final guiding principle is this. Arrange for children to develop their thinking in concrete situations but, above all, allow them plenty of time for this. Half-formed concepts are elusive – they still require verbal support and are easily forgotten. Dyslexic children need to be able *to complete* their learning with concrete materials and we have to create the opportunities for them to do so.

SOME TEACHING EXAMPLES

I have found these basic ideas extremely useful, especially for children who puzzle us because they persistently forget despite years of careful teaching and every opportunity to learn.

I would like to illustrate them with examples of things that work for me. Most of the children I describe attend our dyslexia workshop on a Saturday. We work chiefly on reading and spelling, and tackle mathematics only if children are having persistent difficulty at school.

I usually work with parent and child together. I devise the concrete learning situation beforehand and decide on the language to accompany it. We develop this in the lesson and once it is going smoothly the parent takes over. If everything goes well, they take the kit of materials home and practise during the week. The language is always carefully written down and they both agree to keep to it. This allows a great deal of unhurried talking and manipulating to take place and provides the *time* that children need.

In school, learning situations can be devised in which children work in pairs. The 'Shrink-A-Square' game was designed with this in mind. The teacher sets up the activity, develops the language and then leaves the children to continue on their own.

Once the concept is fully established, it is followed by formal written practice in the usual way. From time to time, I ask children to 'talk their way through' an operation or to explain why a particular step is necessary. This keeps alive the original language and understanding, and maintains links with the concrete stage of the learning.

Teaching addition with carrying to Gemma

Gemma worked on a large plastic-covered board marked in 'tens' and 'units' columns (Figure 3.1), and wrote on it with a black wipe-off pen. She set out an addition sum with Dienes blocks and then I asked:

> 'How many tens have you in the tens position?'
> 'Two.' Gemma pointed to them.
> 'Write it down.' She wrote '2' next to the two rods.
> 'How many units have you in the units position?'
> 'Seven.' Gemma wrote '7' next to the seven units, and we dealt with each number in this way.

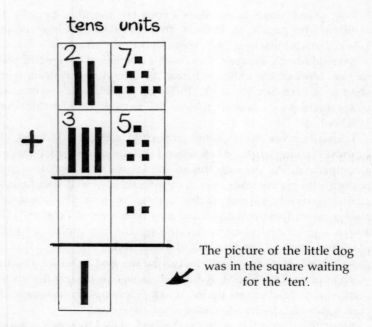

The picture of the little dog was in the square waiting for the 'ten'.

Figure 3.1 Addition with carrying

There was no explanation as such, but Gemma was developing a feel for the fact that '2' written in the tens-position meant two tens, and that '7' in the units-position meant seven units. She was able to *see* the Dienes blocks and figures juxtaposed, repeatedly, through countless exercises, and was strengthening her grasp of the place system.

Gemma had already done some addition using straws. She was used to putting an elastic band around ten straws to make 'one bundle' and moving it across to the tens-position. So in this game, when the units came to more than nine, she 'exchanged 10 units for one ten', and . . .

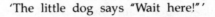

'The little dog says "Wait here!"'

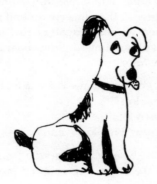

She put the 'ten' under the line in the square with the little dog, and there it remained while she added up the rest of her tens. I gave no explanation for this, but made sure we joked continually about the little dog wanting the 'ten' to wait with him. And as he looked up appealingly from the bottom of the page, I could feel him making his point in Gemma's mind!

The transfer to the formal algorithm was smooth and required no further explanation. Gemma always put the figure she carried under the line, working confidently from the understanding she had gained from the manipulating stage of the learning. She always carried the correct figure, having mentally exchanged her units, and she always remembered where it had to 'wait'.

The language we carefully practised and overlearned was this:

'How many tens have you in the tens-position?'
'How many units have you in the units-position?'
'I need to exchange 10 units for one ten.'

The little dog was used to strengthen a feel for position without needing to explain things in words.

Multiplication – teaching the initial concept to Daniel

To beginners, the language used in multiplication can be confusing. If we say 'three threes are nine', the second 'three' means '3', but the first means something quite different – it means '3 lots of'.

To introduce this idea in a direct non-verbal way, I played a game with bright multicoloured map-pins on a cork floor-tile. I tipped a heap of pins on the table, and while they were still rolling around we each picked up three of the same colour and put them in a row on our cork boards. Then we made another row in a different colour. As we worked away, building up our boards, I developed the language along these lines:

'How many lots of three have you made, Daniel?'
'How many pink lots?'
'How many green lots?'
'Let's make another blue lot' – and so on.

When we had filled the boards, we played a game called 'STOP-ME'. I said, 'Daniel, stop me when I've counted *four* lots of three', and slowly counted the rows of pins.

'One, two, three . . . four, five, six . . .'

Daniel had to shout 'Stop!' as soon as I reached 12 but before I had time to sneak quickly on to 13. I counted rhythmically, quietly stressing 3, 6, 9, 12, and Daniel followed with his finger ready to shout 'Stop!' at just the right moment. To do this, he had to judge what '4 lots of 3' meant on his board and follow carefully while I counted. As he did so, he could *see* the 'lots of 3' as we built up the pattern. He was developing a feel for multiplication in his own way, without any explanation from me.

When this became easy, we swapped roles and Daniel did the counting. We counted quickly now, slightly emphasizing the key numbers at the end of each line. The 3× table was beginning to form. The words were tied to the rows of coloured pins and the number sequence was developing in a concrete situation.

Once 'lots of' was fixed, I alternated it with 'three threes' and finally introduced the more formal language and the symbol. For a long time Daniel used his map-pin board for calculations which required the 3× table, and for a long time the words 'lots of' were regularly alternated with the symbol '×' on my workcards. Gradually, the number sequence became internalized and he was able to work on his own, but whenever he got stuck he still went back to his well-worn board and counted the rows of pins.

By getting Daniel to use his map-pins over a very long period of time, I was able to ensure that the concept of multiplication was formed from a strong concrete base.

Long multiplication and division – with Kathy

Kathy is a bright and cheerful 13-year-old. 'If you can teach Kathy to multiply', her father said, 'I'll be very surprised. All her teachers have tried!'

Kathy could not multiply if it meant going beyond her table square:

'2 × 13?   I haven't a *clue*!'
'Division?   Oh, that's *IMPOSSIBLE*!!'

Kathy's difficulty was not the concepts. She understood exactly what was needed. It was remembering the sequence of operations in the complicated formal procedures that was 'impossible'.

The breakthrough came when we worked with large figures written on cards which were physically moved around and discussed. We worked on a large piece of white formica and scribbled and drew arrows with black dry-wipe pens. Kathy made overlapping cards like this:

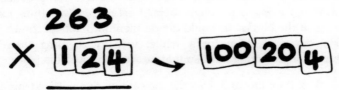

The numbers could be taken apart in layers as she multiplied by each one in turn, and then reassembled at the end as she explained to me why the final addition was necessary.

In division, we worked on a similar scale, but with piles of Dienes blocks instead of numbers. The remainders were 'exchanged' (with appropriate language) for ten smaller blocks, and the whole procedure accompanied by a lively flow of verbal labelling.

Dyslexics have difficulty with sequencing. In mathematics, the algorithms are often long sequences of fairly meaningless operations, and these usually have to be memorized *in words*. Children forget. They mix operations. They often resort to rows of tiny dots and tally marks in an attempt to find a way around the difficulty.

By working in this large multisensory way and developing an understanding of each process, Kathy was able to master these two complex algorithms so that they eventually became easy and fluent. If she forgets, she can draw on her kinesthetic and visual memory of what she did, as well as her knowledge of why each step is necessary. The need to rely on a sequence of verbal instructions has been reduced.

Division – teaching the initial concept to Robert

I was introducing the concept of division to Robert who is 11. His tables book was a mystery to him and he needed the concrete experience of division before we could begin. Young children will happily 'share' sweets among their Teddies and develop understanding in this way. With older children it is difficult. We tried 'sharing' beans in saucers, but this idea was too weak to grip his attention and it did not work.

The answer was to raise the level of difficulty so that it became a challenge and involved his full powers of concentration. I gave him a bag containing 25 wooden blocks and asked him to take out 12 and put them on the table in a row. Once Robert had set them up, he was not allowed to touch them. I asked him whether, just by looking at the blocks, he could divide them into 'lots of three'.

He stared at them for a while, visually dividing them into groups, concentrating hard so that he wouldn't lose his place:

'Yes! It's 4 lots of 3. Exactly!' he said, with a note of triumph in his voice.

We continued, Robert taking from the bag larger and larger handfuls of blocks as he felt he could cope with the challenge. He moved to more difficult tasks. There were 15 blocks set out on the table and I asked,

'How many 4's are there, and what's left over?'
'How many other ways can you divide them?'

Robert was not allowed to touch – however large the number of blocks. He gripped the edge of the table and his hands had to stay there! A fusion of number language and its concrete counterpart was there, and the level of concentration was high. Robert not only grasped the idea of division and remainder but internalized a useful range of number facts as well.

Later, he achieved significant moments like this. There were 18 blocks lined up on the table. Robert studied them carefully and announced:

'6 lots of 3 ...' long pause '... 9 lots of 2'

Then he hesitated, looked excited, thought around in his mind, looked at the wall beyond the blocks and, after several moments of wild thought, said with great delight,

'I know ... I know ... it's 3 lots of SIX as well!'

The exciting thing for me was that Robert didn't look at the blocks at all. He looked at the wall *beyond* while he was deliberating. He seemed to be working from an internal model that was beginning to form – presumably as a result of the high level of concentration needed in order to solve the problems visually.

Once the concept of division was established, we linked the blocks with his tables book. Each time he divided a set of blocks visually, he looked up the result in the relevant table. Gradually the mysteries of the tables book were revealed and we progressed to more formal work from there!

Robert had mastered division but he had also learned a useful range of number facts as well. I feel that tasks similar to this could be devised to help dyslexic youngsters improve their sense of number. The key ingredients appear to be – a fusion of number language with its concrete counterpart combined with a high level of challenge and concentration.

More advanced concepts – with Jonathan

Jonathan and his mother sat down for a lesson. 'I know you want to do the "ough" words today', his mother said, 'but you'll have to help us with Jonathan's Maths homework. We stayed up for hours last night trying to explain $2n + 1 = 9$ but he just can't see what the "n" means!'

I set out a problem with Dienes blocks and hid two blocks in a little plastic box as part of the sum.

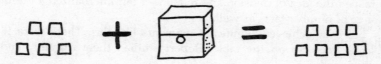

'How many blocks are there in the box?'

Jonathan smiled. There were obviously two. I set up a second problem.... But this time he held back, his eyes thoughtfully dwelling on the blocks and his mind on something else. Then he quickly solved my problem and from then on insisted on setting problems for *us* to solve instead. And very ingenious they were! He quickly introduced '2n' (these were 2 boxes) and then explored the possibilities of different amounts in each box, these were labelled 'n' and 'm'. Soon, he was confidently doing his homework without needing any extra help from us at all.

We had not actually taught Jonathan anything. From the moment I set out the first problem in blocks he took over. He explored the idea himself by inventing problems for us to solve and then quietly got on with his homework without any apparent difficulty. He seemed to have no trouble grasping the relationships once these were made more concrete.

On a similar occasion, he was unable to solve problems to do with angles in a circle.

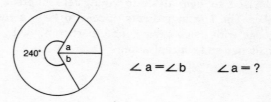

Jonathan knew there were 360 degrees in a circle but he could not see what to do with the 240. His parents had gone to great lengths trying to explain but he seemed unwilling to accept this. Perhaps, like other dyslexics, he had learnt that unless he understood what he was doing it was no good – he would eventually forget. So because he was unable to see where the 240 fitted in, he could not simply accept their explanation as another child might do.

I had planned to tackle this with lentils. It was a rather homespun analogy but it was all that I could think of at the time! I tipped some lentils into a saucer and asked Jonathan to count out 360, very roughly, and spread them in a circle. This took him quite a while. I had intended to take out a sector from the circle and develop the explanation from there, but Jonathan stopped me. He had *seen* what to do. It was obvious, and he wanted to get on with his homework straightaway.

The questions progressed quite quickly in difficulty, covering a range of problems involving general angle properties. Jonathan worked quietly on his own. Occasionally his eyes strayed to the lentils as if seeking support, but the problems were quite clear to him and he required no extra help from us.

It was as though he could not 'think' 360 degrees – this was too intangible. But he could think in terms of lentils and counting out 360 lentils was enough to make the problem sufficiently concrete for him to grasp. This was all he needed. From then on everything fell into place and he was able to continue on his own.

The Dienes blocks in '2n + 1 = 9' had played a similar role. In both these situations Jonathan's ability to understand mathematical relationships was good. What he could not do so well was grasp them in a purely abstract way. He needed concrete support.

As a dyslexic child gets older, he may not need to develop new concepts in concrete situations in the way that younger children do. But the weakness in verbal thinking may still be there. If he asks for help, explaining to him *in words* may only make things worse and add to his confusion. It may be better to present the problem in a concrete form and allow him to see the relationships in this way.

Making symbols meaningful

> 'X' is linked to 'lots of' which in turn is linked to the rows of pins . . .

I would like to end with a tale about young Gemma and her fear of symbols. Gemma had built up her 3X table with map-pins (described above for Daniel) and was familiar with the phrase 'lots of' and the formal symbol 'X'.

She was working through a computer program in which 'lots of' was gradually juxtaposed with the symbol and then finally replaced by it altogether. She would work away quite happily until the symbol 'X' first appeared on the screen. Each time the symbol appeared she quietly walked away from the computer and did something else. And if we attempted to explain the symbol, she very politely changed the subject!

What to do? Gemma, her mother and I played a simple game. We sat in a circle and I asked her, 'What's 2 lots of 3?' 'Six!' Then Gemma asked her mother, 'What's 3 lots of 3?' 'Nine', and so on. Each time we said 'lots of' we crossed our arms in the shape of a multiplication sign. It took the form of a children's song-and-gesture game. We linked the words 'lots of' to the *feel* of a diagonal cross. Then we drew them with coloured pens and called them 'lots of' signs. This worked. The next time Gemma tackled the computer program she responded to the symbol without a murmur!

Gemma showed the same evasive fear for the symbol for division, but I was prepared this time. On our large hand-written worksheets we did this – at the end of each page I asked her to find all the words 'divide' and turn the two dots into big round ones by going over them with a pen. This was fun. They got bigger and bigger and then became brightly coloured. By the time we got to the sixth sheet the dots were an all-important part of the work.

The link between:

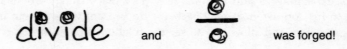

CONCLUSION

In this chapter, I have tried to show that, because of a generalized weakness in language, dyslexic children may have difficulty acquiring mathematical concepts in the normal way. It may be easier for them if they are allowed to explore new ideas with concrete materials and develop their understanding in this way.

This means that in a mathematics class a dyslexic youngster will have different needs. He may be tackling the same work as the other children, yet still require the kind of concrete support we usually associate with a much younger or less able child.

All the children I have described had had years and years of careful patient teaching. It was puzzling how quickly they forgot. We felt that yet more explanation followed by the usual written practice was unlikely to work. We would simply be repeating what had gone before.

Instead, we created opportunities for them to develop their thinking with concrete materials and we strengthened the language they would need. This seems to have helped – and the understanding that is released by this change of approach has surprised us all.

Notes

The Open University course EM235 'Developing Mathematical Thinking' is a good way to begin to explore the ideas developed here. The course is due to be replaced in 1992 by a revised course EM236. Details can be obtained from The Centre for Mathematics Education, The Open University, Milton Keynes, MK7 6AA.

I am grateful to Chris Weeks, my former Open University tutor, for reading this chapter and providing helpful suggestions.

1. Dienes blocks are used in most primary schools and are obtainable from the main educational suppliers.

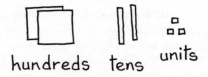

hundreds   tens   units

2. 'Developing Mathematical Thinking', Course EM235, The Open University.
3. 'Embedded' – I use this term in the sense intended by Margaret Donaldson in her book *Children's Minds*, London, Fontana, 1978.

Chapter 4

Reading and writing in mathematics

Elaine Miles

To speak of dyslexic children having 'mathematical' difficulties may obscure the fact that many of these difficulties are of a linguistic nature and are therefore not unexpected in view of their particular weaknesses in the literacy field. There are a great many different points at which such weaknesses may affect their mathematics, and my chief object in this chapter is to survey them, although occasionally I may briefly suggest some way of helping.

DIFFICULTIES WITH THE TEXT OF A PROBLEM

The first thought that springs to mind, given the title of this chapter, is that dyslexic children may be handicapped in reading the text of problems. If an ordinary situation is being described, such as building a bookcase or papering the walls of a room, a certain level of reading skill is assumed; and it may be extra hard for the dyslexic if the setter attempts to make the problem interesting by choosing less everyday objects as the subjects of the problem, for example by asking the price of a number of 'embroidery skeins' instead of 'pencils' or by asking how long it will take to drive from Avignon to Chalons at a given speed rather than from Leeds to Bradford – since these pose extra decoding puzzles. The dyslexic may also be bothered by longer unfamiliar words chosen to give greater mathematical precision, such as 'dimensions' used instead of 'size'.

Perhaps less obvious a difficulty is the fact that the approach to reading required is not that to which he is accustomed, although this may not have been made clear by his teachers. He is perhaps practised in getting the gist of a story (and in the present climate of opinion in reading instruction is probably encouraged to do so). Being used, then, to concentrate on what is happening he is now, on the contrary, expected to ignore the narrative and look for relationships. Having read the problem through and perhaps been reminded of the bookcase at home or of the time when his father papered the hall, in the examples I suggested earlier, he may be no nearer understanding what sort of sum is needed because he is not focusing on the right things. In this situation, to draw a picture of the bookcase or the room may help him to pick out the essentials of what is required. Another helpful device is for him to rewrite the question in his own words.

It is common practice to tell a child, when tackling a problem, to look first to see what is 'given'. However, what is 'given' will be found in small details scattered around the text, just like those 'little words' which in his previous reading experience he has been most accustomed to overlook, for example

45 cm, 54°

Labelling the picture which he has drawn will force him to go back and look at these details carefully.

The style of a sentence in a mathematical problem is often tortuous and condensed, and therefore difficult to construe, for example

'The perimeter of a rectangular piece of paper is 4.8 cm.'

Brief and to the point? However, the first thing that we need to pick out is that it is a *rectangular* piece of paper; only then is the word 'perimeter' meaningful. Yet the word 'rectangular' is buried in the middle of the sentence.

There is also a major difficulty about vocabulary. In all his reading in mathematics, not only of problems, but also of the explanations which he finds in his class mathematics book, he will find a plethora of technical terms, since each new topic brings a fresh collection of them. They are of two types: there are the ones which are deceptively familiar but used in a quite different sense from the one that he associates with them, and there are the much more lengthy ones which are totally new.

Examples of the first type are the following, with the associations that the child is likely to bring to them:

makes   (mother makes a cake)

take away   (Chinese take-away)

odd	(something peculiar)
even	(keep your handwriting even)
set	(tea-set)
square	(meet me in the square)
power	(there's been a power cut)
division	(Liverpool is in the first division)
dividend	(what Dad hopes to get from the pools)
index	(look it up at the back of the book)
compass	(take it with you on Dartmoor)
vulgar	(!)
improper	(!)

In everyday life these words either have much less exact meanings than those demanded by their mathematical use, or may even have totally different associations; either way confusion is likely. The town square that the child knows is of indefinite shape; food bought at a 'Chinese take-away' is totally removed, and taking always involves discrete objects. The concept of 'division' as a mathematical operation is far from the thoughts of a young football fan. Such vivid associations are not easily dispelled merely by rote learning of phrases, for example 'An even number is one which is divisible by two.' In this case the terms 'even number' and 'odd number' may need to be illustrated spatially for the full implications to be seen by a child who naturally thinks in spatial terms, perhaps in some such way as this (Figure 4.1):

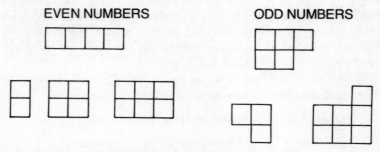

Figure 4.1 Spatial illustration of even and odd numbers

Even the words 'write/right' may be a source of confusion, as reported by one who was herself a dyslexic (Street 1976):

> Write it down.
> You haven't got it right.
> Put the 1 right up at the top.
> Now make that right.
> Put it on the right.
> Right, now we'll do another one.

The second set of mathematical terms are those which are likely to appear quite alien to the child, and the relevance of the underlying concept to the sums involved is quite likely not to be grasped at all. Such words become difficult for the dyslexic to remember in detail and therefore to spell; nor are they of any use to him in performing the mathematical operations.
Examples are:

numerator	quadrilateral	quotient
denominator	simultaneous	vector
isosceles	proportion	coefficient
hypotenuse	binary	ratio

How, for instance, is one supposed to remember which term is which of 'numerator' and 'denominator', even with a classical education to help with the derivations? Yet one may perfectly understand, without using these terms, what the top and bottom numbers in a fraction each stand for. The word 'isosceles' is particularly puzzling. No word that the child has ever met has either of the parts of the word 'isosceles' , 'iso-', or 'scel-', to help him determine how to spell it. A correspondence in *The Times* on the subject resulted in a list of 270 different ways of spelling this word from the work of schoolchildren. We treasure the list which was sent to us by Brian Cook who was responsible for collecting most of them. Here are a few examples which illustrate the point well. Most are phonetically acceptable.

aesosaleis	isosalise	oisossilies
aysosalease	isosyles	nicoselise
hysosiles	issossiloese	nysosalis

Two of these examples ('nicoselise' and 'nysosalis') presumably come from children who did not appreciate where words divided in 'an isosceles triangle'. An extra complication about this word is that in talking about *all three* sides being equal the term 'equilateral' is used, but when we want to say that *two* sides are equal we have to use another word from a different root; yet 'iso-' and 'equi-' in fact mean the same thing! Virtually all the words in my second list (the unfamiliar technical terms) have no word in common use from the same root to compare for spelling purposes.

I remember the word 'proportion' causing terrible trouble for one pupil whom I taught. She professed to be unable to do 'proportion' sums at all and asked to have them explained to her. In a practical situation, away from the terminology, working out how much five pencils will cost when seven cost 28p seems simple enough, and I came to the conclusion that it was the technical term which was blinding her to the obvious. Using more technical terms than necessary is putting obstacles in the way of understanding for the dyslexic. Perhaps we should consider which are essential.

Finally there is the problem that the same operation may be signalled by a large variety of everyday terms. Thus 'altogether', 'total', 'sum', 'plus', 'add' and 'and' must all equally be interpreted as 'addition sum needed here', while – perhaps even more perplexing – 'minus', 'difference', and 'how much more?' must all be taken to mean 'do a subtraction sum'. They are all being used as technical terms, although they do not appear to be. The child probably needs to be specifically alerted to the range of expressions like this that will indicate to him what he has to *do* when he starts to think in terms of sums.

DIFFICULTIES WITH THE SYMBOLIC LANGUAGE OF MATHEMATICS

The arabic numerals

So far we have been talking only about difficulties associated with use of the alphabetic symbolization which the child has met in his reading books. But mathematics has its own symbolic language, which has to be learned. For the dyslexic, pushing numbers about without understanding their function will prove no more successful than pushing letters about when he was dealing with the alphabet, and will result in similar muddles with their order and in possible confusion between those of similar visual appearance, for example 5 and 8.

Position is even more important in mathematics than it is in spelling. Whereas the teacher may possibly guess that you mean 'brain' when you write 'brian', because the latter is not a noun of wide application and needs a capital letter to be meaningful, it is not likely that she will realize that you mean '1,438' when you write '1,348'; and when the error has been compounded by addition or subtraction there is total chaos. Although nowadays in the early stages of mathematics teachers are encouraged to do practical work with concrete objects to give the basis for number concepts, this may not have been enough for the dyslexic, or may have come at too early a stage for him to learn from it. He is then pushed on with the others to doing *what the teacher tells him to do* without having grasped why. This is especially true of carrying figures. Teacher tells him to put a little figure 1 at the top, so he does. Henceforward he expects any little working number at the top to be a 1.

Small differences in the position of numbers are also sometimes used to mark important distinctions in mathematics. Consider these series, which are given in a cheap book of 'Home Tests' – part of a so-called intelligence test:

22. 1. 2. 3. 4.
23. 1. 4. 7. 10.
24. 3. 4. 6. 9.
25. 35. 30. 25. 20.

The child has to continue the series. He must be careful to realise that the first number is the number of the question and therefore not to be included, especially in the fourth case, where it is tempting to do so. A clearly laid out page is particularly important for the dyslexic. Another source of bewilderment is the important differences signalled by size and position, for example

$$23 \qquad 22.3 \qquad 22^3 (10648) \qquad 22_3(8)$$

The symbolization of fractions is something particularly difficult to grasp, because numbers in fractions cannot be treated exactly the same way as whole numbers, but this is not always realized. Consequently the dyslexic will readily use an inappropriate algorithm, as in this example given to me once by a teacher in New Zealand (Figure 4.2).

$$\frac{5}{6} - \frac{1}{3} = \frac{2}{12} - \frac{5}{12} = \frac{3}{12}$$

$$\frac{7}{8} - \frac{3}{4} = \frac{3}{16} - \frac{5}{16} = \frac{3}{16}$$

$$\frac{8}{9} - \frac{1}{2} = \frac{6}{18} - \frac{8}{18} = \frac{2}{18}$$

Figure 4.2 The symbolization of fractions

In fact the girl has used a consistent method throughout, but it was one appropriate to cancellation of factors rather than subtraction. For having chosen a common denominator perfectly correctly (even if at times an unnecessarily high one) she then did a subtraction sum diagonally between the numerator of one fraction and the denominator of the other, in either direction, rather as one does when dividing by common factors. The working, on that principle, is perfectly correct.

Particular difficulties will also arise from the dyslexic's confusion over direction and his general inflexibility of approach. In following a text in a reading book, the pupil has been taught to move from left to right. In mathematics he must be flexible, depending on the operation required. If he understands base 10 properly because of having had experience with concrete materials, he will appreciate that in doing addition and multiplication sums he must do the right-hand column first because he may have to 'trade' if he has more than 10, and these 'tens' need to be included in the next column to the left when he gets to it. (He will understand that, because previously he will have found himself in a position of having to go back again if he went the wrong way as he worked with blocks.) A dyslexic child has to understand explicitly in a way that may not be necessary for the more linguistically able members of the class, who simply accept that they have to work in a particular direction.

In dealing with an equation, on the other hand, the mathematical equivalent of a sentence, he must be prepared to read it from left to right *or* right to left according to what he needs to do. If, for instance, this pupil has always read:

$6 + 4 =$ what?

and never:

what $- 4 = 6$?

or:

$10 -$ what $= 6$?

which would train him to see how these operations are inter-changeable, he will not be able to 'juggle about' with figures – for example using the commutative principle to make multiplication sums easier; thus:

3×7 is the same as 7×3

He may be unsure about the $7\times$ table but completely confident about the $3\times$ table. This is very important for the dyslexic, for whom multiplication tables are a major source of difficulty.

Algebraic symbols

This flexibility is very important for algebra. The dyslexic may be completely at a loss what to do when he sees:

$x - 5 = 16$

unless of course he can recognize it as the same type of sentence as the one he met earlier:

what $- 5 = 16$?

Both are in effect asking 'What number can you take 5 from and leave 16?' Dyslexics are not alone in having difficulty in coping with equations, but they are particularly vulnerable to this sort of difficulty where the task demands flexibility and a sense of direction.

There are also other problems with algebraic notation. Algebraic equations are often a shorthand way of saying two things at once and these have to be separated out and dealt with in turn; thus:

$3x - 5 = 16$

is saying *both* that a number is 5 more than 16 *and* that the number that we are really seeking is a third of that number. The pupil has to understand that $3x$ is itself a number, which has to be worked out first.

The notation for such numbers is also different from the arithmetical one. Thirty-five means three tens and five units, but 3x means three times x; with algebraic symbols multiplication signs are not used – the number and the algebraic symbol are just put next to each other. Similarly (a+b)(a+b) means (a+b) times (a+b), with the bracket holding the complex number together. Such a complex expression is very difficult to understand, but a spatially-inclined pupil may understand it perfectly if shown a diagram like the following (Figure 4.3) which illustrates (a+b)(a+b) as representing an area of an enlarged square, originally with a side of length 'a', to which has been added an extension in each direction of length 'b' to form a square of side 'a+b'. It is easy then to see how the new total area is expressed by $a^2 + 2ab + b^2$, the sum of the area of four different pieces.

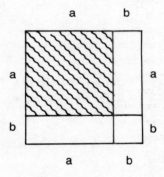

Figure 4.3 Spatial illustration of (a + b)(a + b)

Dienes (1960) uses just such a method to demonstrate the meaning of algebraic concepts.

Even at a more sophisticated level there is always the difficulty of understanding how a symbol for a variable differs from a symbol acting as a name. A striking example of this is given by Mestre and Gerace (1986) in a question which they set to bilingual students who might be expected to have additional language problems:

> Mr Smith noted the number of cars, C, and the number of trucks, T, in a parking lot and wrote the following equation to represent the situation:
>
> 8C=T

Are there more cars or trucks in this parking lot? Why?

One would expect this problem to bother others besides dyslexics, but it is an illustration of symbols being used in different ways, alphabetically and mathematically. 'C' and 'T' do not stand for 'cars' and 'trucks', but for the *numbers* of cars and trucks respectively. They are variables, not names.

Mathematical symbols other than numerals

Here the first ones which spring to mind are the ones which the child meets first, namely $+$, $-$, $\times$, $\div$, and $=$. Many mistakes are made if the first four are not clearly differentiated. It is probably valuable to explain the relationship between addition and multiplication and the relationship between subtraction and division; these are represented by the fact that the two symbols in each pair look more like each other, in each case the second one being a development from its partner. Understanding of these relationships and of the contrasting opposition of the two pairs to each other makes it more easy to remember which is which.

Difficulty over direction often gets dyslexics into trouble over the signs for 'greater than' and 'less than', namely $>$ and $<$. Although others may just *remember* to draw the sign from left to right for 'more than' and the other way for 'less than', the dyslexic needs to be taught to recognize both as static figures between two numbers, with the wide 'mouth' facing the larger number, and the tiny point next to the small number, for example

$$5 < 8$$

$$6 > 4$$

Put that way, direction does not come into it.

These are only two of the large number of extra symbols, in addition to the arabic numerals, which the budding mathematician has to learn, involving a far greater burden of paired associate learning than in learning the use of the alphabet. Mathematics also constantly makes other nice distinctions represented by tiny differences in the symbol used, for example different sorts of brackets, round, curly and straight, used in different areas of mathematics:

$$( ) \quad \{ \} \quad [ ]$$

There are also the hoop-like symbols used in set theory to denote membership of classes. I find it particularly to the point that in a popular series of books on mathematics foundation skills for 11- to 14-year olds there is a cartoon in which a boy is gazing at some shelf brackets and the teacher is saying 'not *that* sort of brackets!'.

If we take into account how in these many different ways linguistic facility is needed in the building of basic arithmetical skills, we shall apply some of the same techniques in helping dyslexics with their mathematics that we do in teaching them literacy skills; that is we have to make quite clear what function the symbols are performing, without taking anything for granted.

It is, of course, quite true that children other than dyslexics may suffer from some of the difficulties which I have mentioned. What is important is that we separate out the linguistic components of mathematical difficulties and deal with them explicitly when that is needed. As we know, dyslexics are particularly vulnerable in linguistic areas.

Let me end with an example given by a dyslexic (Street 1976) of the confusion caused mainly by what the teacher is *saying* to her. The author uses capitals to indicate the words over which she had to stop and think.

We are going to TAKE 25 FROM 61. WRITE DOWN 61 first (I sometimes wrote the first figure I heard before the second one.) WRITE DOWN 25 UNDERNEATH it. Put the 2 UNDER the 6 and the 5 UNDER the 1. Draw a line UNDERNEATH. Start at the bottom on the RIGHT. Take 5 AWAY FROM 1. It won't go. Start again. Borrow 10 FROM the 6. (Confusion here because you take smaller numbers from bigger ones, and 10 take away 6 is 4.) 'Where do I put the 4?' There isn't a 4 in the sum. Now pay attention ... start again. You are borrowing 10 FROM 60. (Confusion again because that seems to leave a 50 somewhere). You borrow the 10 from the 60 and add it to the 1 to make 11. Then you take the 5 AWAY FROM 11. That leaves 6. Put the 6 DOWN, UNDER the line BELOW the 5. There is no need to take so long. Take the one you have borrowed AWAY FROM the 6. 'Which 6?'. Then take 2 AWAY FROM the 6. 'Which 6?'. Then take 2 AWAY FROM 5. That leaves 3. If you like you can pay back the 10 to the 2 and that makes 3. Then you take 3 AWAY FROM 6, and you get the same answer, 3. Put the 3 DOWN, on the LEFT of the 6. Not that 6, the one in your answer. Read the answer from LEFT to RIGHT – 36.

Eventually Street taught herself to subtract by her own private method (which involved adding), despite the disapproval of her teacher who said that this method was too confusing!

REFERENCES

Dienes, Z.P. (1960) *Building up Mathematics*, London, Hutchinson Educational.

Mestre, J. and Gerace, W. (1980) 'The interplay of linguistic factors in mathematical translation tasks', *Focus on Learning Problems in Mathematics* 8 (1), 59–72.

Street, J. (1976) 'Sequencing and directional confusion in arithmetic', *Dyslexia Review* 15, 16–19.

Chapter 5

Difficulties at the secondary stage

Anne Henderson

INTRODUCTION

According to Steeves (1983) and Joffe (1981) many dyslexics have much potential to succeed in mathematics once they have grasped the basic concepts. In fact some dyslexics are capable of scaling great heights with their mathematical prowess. With this in mind a teacher should never underestimate potential and should try to ensure that opportunities for advanced goals are available should students want them. Once a concept is mastered fully, to ask a pupil to complete pages and pages of similar problems is a waste of time. He should be given the chance to move on.

DEALING WITH THE TENSION

Fear and anxiety associated with mathematics are often magnified in a dyslexic pupil. In the case of my own work, which is mostly with dyslexics aged between 11 and 16, at first, I regularly see them in a one-to-one teaching situation; and if they do not know me they may well conclude that their 'stupidity' (as they see it) will be exposed. Even though many of them will have been told that they are *not* just 'stupid' they may still be lacking in confidence and be unable to shake off the belief that they are going to fail. I once had a pupil who came to me, white-faced and stiff-backed, who proceeded to grip the pencil with hot sweaty hands, and who showed not just fear but sheer panic. A first lesson in this atmosphere is a tough experience for pupil and teacher alike.

To be effective in this kind of situation a teacher needs to have confidence in her own abilities to help. This in turn enhances the pupil's confidence. Encouraging the pupil to talk about himself and to discuss the way he sees his maths problem is a good way of beginning a working relationship. Allowing the pupil to mention past failures and incidents that have embarrassed him with regard to his dyslexia is a way of improving this relationship.

It also helps if the pupil and teacher can discuss a topic common to both of them, possibly a school trip, a school activity, or even some outside event with which they are both familiar. Games may help to ease the atmosphere, since the emphasis is not so much on the pupil as on playing the game, and this is a way of taking the pressure out of a one-to-one situation. Using a game to start a lesson heightens a pupil's awareness of number and also helps to prevent any anxiety he may feel about his lack of ability at the subject. Allowing a pupil to discuss and talk freely about his problems gives him the opportunity to express and to show his own strengths and weaknesses. Humour, too, is something that eases anxious moments and enables the pupil to relax.

It is necessary to identify the place where the pupil is in his mathematics education and to start helping him there. The teacher should observe the pupil to see his reactions to certain mathematical topics. Having long-term goals with short-term objectives can be helpful. Dyslexic children are difficult to assess, since the pace at which they move through a topic may vary, and some have an extraordinary potential to 'see' answers or develop strategies for coping.

Pupils who have a specific difficulty are also individuals with their own learning style (compare this book, Chapter 2). It is interesting to observe the methods which they use and, where appropriate, to incorporate improvements. If pictorial or verbal mnemonics, or material on tape, help a student to learn a particular mathematical point, then the teacher should try to make sure that these are available as much as possible. Once a pupil finds a method by which he learns, his self-esteem is enhanced and he will have the confidence to make good progress.

When dealing with a dyslexic pupil the teacher should be fully conversant with the effect that his language difficulties are having on his mathematics. In the knowledge that sequencing and direction problems and problems of short-term memory will all be contributing to the pupil's learning difficulties, a teacher should be continually on the look-out for problematic areas and be ready to help with ideas and suggestions. Identification of a problem is not easy, but if a teacher is aware of its existence she can be on the alert. Emphasizing strengths is not new to teaching; but when a pupil has failed many times it is vitally important to build up confidence by telling him – and showing him – that he is able to do something well. Even winning a little game and beating the teacher is enough to start a growth of self-esteem. Encouraging his success and calling attention to work that has been well done will contribute further to promoting his confidence.

EXAMPLES OF DIFFICULTIES

Sometimes the pupil will discuss correctly the method that he has used. Then several problems are worked through orally, and he will go through each stage step by step, showing clearly that he understands the concept. Even when a slightly different calculation arises he will deal with it quite competently and tell the teacher exactly what needs to be done. Yet, when it comes to doing the calculation, even with the aid of a calculator, he comes up with the wrong answer. The teacher discusses the method once more; the computation is repeated – and the answer is wrong again! The teacher will eventually discover that, although the pupil is *saying* the correct word, for example, 'multiply', he will be constantly pressing the 'divide' button on the calculator. This sends the whole calculation wrong. The following is an example of precisely this mistake:

One of my pupils, Bob, aged 14, was given the following question:

A factory worker earns a basic pay of £3.20 an hour for a 36-hour week. For any extra hours he is paid time and a half. Calculate his earnings if he works for 39 hours.

This is what he said he would do:

£3.20 for 36 hours = £3.20 × 36 = £115.20
To find time and a half divide the £3.20 by 2 = £1.60
Add this £1.60 to the £3.20 = £4.80
Multiply £4.80 by 3 = £14.40
Total £115.20 + £14.40 = £129.60

But this is what he did:

£3.20 × 36 = £115.20
£3.20 ÷ 2 = £1.60
£1.60 + £3.20 = £4.80

So far so good. But the next step was £4.80 × 3. Here he pressed the ÷ button, and he was so engrossed that he was not aware of this error! Since £4.80 ÷ 3 came to £1.60 he proceeded as follows:

£1.60 + £115.20 = £116.80

The answer was wrong but his understanding of the concepts was entirely correct.

Here is a similar example but at a more advanced level. Mark, aged 15, had been given the following problem in trigonometry:

A triangle, CBN, has angle N the right-angle; angle B is 28°, and the hypotenuse, BC, is 3 metres. What is the length of CN and BN?

Mark drew the triangle correctly; he then thought out the formulae for *sine* and *cosine*, namely that 'sine' is 'opposite over hypotenuse' and 'cosine' is 'adjacent over hypotenuse'. This gave him:

$$\sin 28° = \frac{CN}{3}$$

This gave him that CN was 1.4 metres.

He then repeated the procedure, and wrote:

$$\cos 28° = \frac{BN}{3}$$

When he came to do the calculation, however, *he copied the value of sin 28° over again*! This meant that BN was also 1.4 metres, which was clearly absurd. On these and similar occasions it is worth reminding the pupil that he should not simply equate 'wrong answer' with failure or see the situation simply as another setback. He has in fact gone most of the way towards solving the problem and has understood the important points.

Another difficulty for dyslexics is the recognition of the decimal point within a number. One thing that can go wrong is that the comma dividing off the thousands is often mistaken for the real decimal point. Using a big red plastic decimal point can emphasize its place and also give the pupil a tactile object to reinforce his knowledge. With amounts involving money a pupil may recognize the amount orally but may have difficulty in punching the correct amount into the calculator. Problems arise with values of pounds and single unit pence, for example, £1.06 or £6.07, which the pupil may punch in as '£1.60' or '£6.70'. Also the reverse may happen, so that a reading of £1.6 is read as 'one pound six pence', while £6.7 might be read as 'six pounds seven pence'. Sometimes a pupil will just ignore the decimal point! This can cause considerable trouble especially if the amount involved is only pence, for example, 68p. If the answer needs to be given in pence there is no problem, but if it has to be given in pounds and the student is unaware of his error then he can get into all kinds of difficulties. Here is an example which arose in the case of one of my pupils, David, aged 15.

The problem which he was asked to solve was as follows:

> A man travelled 12,000 miles in a car, buying petrol at a price of 44p per litre. If his car·travelled an average of 11 miles per litre, calculate the estimated cost of the petrol used in the car, giving the correct answer to the nearest whole pound.

David recognized that if he divided 12,000 by 11 it would give the number of litres used, and he also saw that if he multiplied this number by 44p he would get the answer that he needed. He highlighted the symbols so as to clarify the procedures:

$$\div \qquad 12,000 \div 11 = 1090.9091$$
$$\times \qquad 1090.9091 \times 44p$$

He punched in 44 but forgot that the answer was in pence: the man, it seemed, spent £48,000 on petrol each year! At this point David started to panic, realizing that this answer was obviously wrong. Like many others in a stress situation he then came up with a wholly inappropriate suggestion, namely 'Shall I multiply 11 by 44? Will that give me a better answer?'

In such circumstances it is very easy for the teacher to show impatience or at least disappointment. What is needed may in fact be an encouraging smile or a 'Don't worry', since these will help him to relax. Teacher and pupil can then work together in discovering where the pupil went wrong and working out strategies which will enable him to avoid similar mistakes in the future. Where a single error leads to an absurd result it is important to remind him that there is nothing wrong with his understanding of what is needed and that if he continues to make occasional errors of this kind this is a tiresome complication but is in no way evidence that he is 'no good at maths'.

Because of the dyslexic's distinctive weaknesses, the symbol/

language connection needs continually to be talked about. Wall charts can be provided, as well as cards which the pupil can carry around with him and use for reference. Any mathematical terms which the pupil will encounter within a particular topic should be discussed and written down before the topic is begun. This can help avoid the anxious moments which can arise if the word is encountered and not understood. Teachers can build up important vocabulary lists with individual pupils, and these can be related not only to mathematics but to other curriculum subjects. A pupil can print out his list on a word processor and can share his work with others. Creating a folder to which all pupils can contribute is often a good idea: it makes an interesting project, and, since it is cross-curricular, enthusiasm may spread to other subjects.

In dealing with fractions, for example, it is useful gradually to introduce the pupil to words connected with the topic, for example 'parts', 'groups', 'divide', 'vulgar', 'improper', 'denominator', 'numerator', and so on. This will be a safeguard against later panic.

There are some dyslexics who are very good at mental arithmetic and are able to work out the answer in double-quick time. However, in the GCSE examination points are given for method. This means that, even though their answer is correct, if they do not record their working they will lose marks. For many pupils writing down a process in little stages is the easy part of a computation; for a dyslexic it is likely to be the part which he finds most difficult. He may give the correct answer – then, when he picks up a pen and begins to write, he crosses out, starts again, swallows hard, gets sweaty hands, makes yet another mistake – and decides that the whole thing is too much for him. In cases such as this it could even be a good idea to tell the pupil to go through the whole paper putting down answers and then come back and begin to record those methods which he is able to explain.

Sometimes in mathematics, if the calculation involves big numbers, fractions or decimal points, the student is shown how to round off the numbers so as to make the computation simpler. Teaching him to use 'easy' numbers – for example numbers without decimal points – can help him to grasp a particular concept more fully. Thus:

$$526.3 \div 47.61$$

might be written as:

500 ÷ 50

Hence the answer is approximately 10. Many dyslexic pupils will see the point of doing the rounding off, discuss the method in detail and agree wholeheartedly with it. But when a problem arises that is slightly different a pupil may be influenced by the differences in wording or presentation of the problem and fail to use the approximated answer properly.

The following was a problem which I gave to William, one of my pupils aged 14:

> 15 pencils are in a pack that is 20 cm wide.
> How thick is each pencil?

I suggested, in the usual way, that it might help him if he thought in terms of simpler numbers in the first place, and I therefore said to him: '3 pencils are in a pack that is 6 cm wide. How thick is each pencil?' He saw that the answer was 2 cm and returned to the original problem. There was a long pause. In my naïvety I was totally bewildered by this. I had, as I thought, shown him quite clearly what do do and could not understand his hesitation. Finally he said to me, 'How can these pencils change width? If they were 2 cm there' (referring to my 'simpler' example), 'how can they be different now?' I realized that instead of clarifying the situation I had actually made it more complicated.

I had a similar experience with Richard, who was aged 16. We were dealing with pie charts when the following problem arose:

> If 360 degrees represent £1,000 what does 1 degree represent?

Richard proceeded to do the following computation:

360 ÷ 1,000 = 0.36

He realized, however, that this was wrong, having estimated that each degree of the 'pie' must have a value of about £3. I therefore tried to help him by using simpler numbers: 'if 10° represents £20 what does 1° represent?' He immediately gave the correct answer, £2, and realized that he had divided the £20 by the number of degrees. He then solved the earlier problem without any trouble. After this, however, we passed on to another problem in which 40° represented 600 cars. Richard then asked, 'How can 1 degree represent 15 cars when' (pointing to 1° = £2) 'we proved that 1 degree was £2?'

This apparent inability to adjust to new situations can cause confusion in many different topics.

A similar point is illustrated in the case of Matthew, who was aged 14. He had been working out the areas of triangles through practical work – by drawing them and by cutting them up to make rectangles; and we had agreed that to find the area of a triangle was in fact very easy since all that was needed was:

½ the base × the height

Matthew seemed very confident and used the formula many times successfully. I thought that he had mastered and understood the concept. However, much later, when we were doing some revision on this same topic, he got into difficulty. Trying to jog his memory I mentioned the practical work that we had done previously and talked about cutting up triangles to find their areas. Matthew said quite emphatically that using the formula 'half base times height' was applicable only when equilateral triangles were involved – that was the only example which he had remembered from the previous work; all the other examples which he had completed successfully had been forgotten.

Transferring a method from one calculation to another seems too much for them to do. Once a method has seemingly been grasped, a pupil will energetically set down the next problem, taking great care to do things properly; then he will exactly copy a part of the previous one which has got absolutely nothing to do with the present one.

Throughout this work the basic difficulties seem to be connected to the four 'operators', '+', '−', '×' and '÷'. At least one and more often two or more are required to complete a computation, and it is essential that the pupil should be able to identify and understand the processes that each one signifies. Although it is plain from the above examples that these four symbols are very important, equally important is the '=' symbol; this is used just as frequently as the others but is rarely talked about.

THE '=' SIGN

Children meet the 'equals' sign early in their education and the language associated with it starts at this stage. They may come across the word 'is', 'the same as', 'means', 'is equivalent to', and so on. Perhaps their first encounter with it is in a simple equation in the infant department:

$$1 + 2 = 3 \qquad \text{or} \qquad 6 - 4 = 2$$

As a pupil progresses through school he may meet the symbol every day in connection, not only with mathematics, but also with other subjects across the curriculum. Eventually he will meet it formally in algebra. At this point the dyslexic child may well feel sure that he will never be able to understand it because by this time letters are causing problems and when they appear in a problem alongside numbers the difficulty is compounded. From observations of older pupils, especially those reaching GCSE levels, it has become apparent that 'understanding' the meaning of an equation is something which they have never managed. Although they have written the symbol is '=' every day for many years its actual mathematical meaning has eluded them. In finding methods of helping individual pupils who are trying to cope with Pythagoras's theorem or trigonometrical ratios but have never been able to manipulate values on different sides of equations a return to basics is essential. The area is one in which the typical difficulties of the dyslexic clearly show themselves.

It is important to check in the first place that the pupil is familiar with some of the basic principles of algebra. These are:

(i)   'x' is the same as '+1x'.
(ii) '2x' means '2 multiply by x',
(iii) a bracket means 'multiply',
(iv) the commutative principle applies to both '+' and '×'. Thus '1 × 2' is the same as '2 × 1' and '1 + 2' is the same as '2 + 1' (but '1 ÷ 2' is not the same as '2 ÷ 1' and '1 − 2' is not the same as '2 − 1').

There are two different ways of explaining how the '=' sign works in the solving of equations. In the first place it can be thought of as a balance which must be kept level at all times. In that case, if something is done to one side of the equation, then precisely the same thing must be done to the other. Secondly, the pupil can be shown how it is that the mathematical symbols all have opposite values when they are moved through the '=' sign on to the opposite side of the equation. Here is an example:

Find the value of x in the following equation:

$$3x - 2 = x + 12$$

If the first method is used a record can be kept of all the things that are done to both sides. The working might then look like this:

Do this to
each side

$$3x - 2 = x + 12$$
$$3x - 2 + 2 = x + 12 + 2 \qquad (+2)$$
$$3x = x + 14$$
$$3x - x = x + 14 - x \qquad (-x)$$
$$2x = 14$$
$$x = 7 \qquad (\div 2)$$

If the second method is used the following principles apply:

$+$ becomes $-$
$-$ becomes $+$
$\times$ becomes $\div$
$\div$ becomes $\times$

We start, as before, with the original equation:

$$3x - 2 = x + 12$$

Then:

-2 becomes $+2$, therefore $\quad 3x = x + 12 + 2$
therefore $\quad 3x = x + 14$
$+x$ becomes $-x$, therefore $\quad 3x - x = 14$
therefore $\quad 2x = 14$
$\times 2$ becomes $\div 2$, therefore $\quad x = 14 \div 2$
therefore $\quad x = 7$

Once the pupil has decided on a method to tackle a problem (whether the first or the second of these methods) he should be allowed to proceed at his own pace without interference.

Various difficulties, however, may show themselves. Thus:

(i) If a pupil has solved an equation successfully by means of the second method (for instance by moving -2 across the equation so that it becomes $+2$), then when he starts to do the next equation he will look back to see how he began the previous one and may copy not only the method but also the actual digits involved.

(ii) He may forget that 2x is '2 times x' and simply take away the 2 to leave x.

(iii) He may forget which symbol is the opposite of the one which he is considering, for instance, by thinking of $-$ as $\div$; or he may be concentrating so hard on remembering which is the 'opposite' that he may forget to move the value to the other side.

(iv) When using the first method he may add 3 to one side and forget to add it to the other.

(v) Sometimes he may connect the symbols '+' and '$-$' to the preceding letter. Thus 3x $-$ x would be read as $-$3x $+$ x

If the teacher is aware of the possible errors and emphasizes the appropriate details it is possible to pre-empt some of these difficulties, even if not all of them. Once a pupil has a good grasp of equations it gives him confidence in other subjects across the curriculum where they occur, such as physics, chemistry and biology. It also means that mathematical formulae, for example, $C = 2\pi r$ or $A = \pi r$, or trigonometrical ratios or time/speed ratios, do not create such anxiety as before because the pupil has acquired several strategies to help him 'find a way' through to solving a problem. Knowing he is able to attack a problem in different ways gives him a flexibility of approach which does not restrict him and which therefore gives him confidence.

One pupil said: 'Now I know a lot of little ways through I try out different ones till I can find the right answer.' Another pupil said: 'Because I know there is not just one way of finding an answer, which I usually can't remember, I search for another method I understand instead of giving up.'

Working with a student who is keen to achieve makes the teacher aware, not only that the lesson must be interesting, but that it must contain material which will stretch the pupil's abilities and make him reach a higher level of achievement. If one is working with pupils with learning difficulties it is very easy to lower one's aims and objectives; and if a pupil thinks that his teacher does not expect him to achieve very much, then there is a tendency for the pupil not to achieve $-$ the low aspirations of the teacher somehow permeate to the pupil.

USE OF CALCULATORS

In most examinations pupils are allowed the use of calculators. However, as has been shown already, they are liable to press the wrong symbol button because the language associated with it has confused them. A most important skill in this connection is estimation. It is necessary not only for checking computational work but in everyday life where exact answers are not necessary or are difficult to obtain.

There are various ways in which estimation can be carried out. Once a pupil begins to understand the concept then different processes can be discussed.

To round off to the nearest 10 or 100 helps the grasp of place value and enables the student to get an answer quickly. Thus:

48 + 43 becomes 50 + 40 = 90

Reading a number on a calculator needs practice. A pupil needs to be shown how to read and correct a number to either significant figures or decimal places. As was mentioned earlier, vocabulary needs to be discussed and written down, and this applies to abbreviations also. Thus 'decimal place' might be written as 'd.pl.', 'significant figures' as 'sig.fig.' or 'S.F.', and 'correct' as 'corr.'

Here are some problems that I have encountered:

(i) *Correct £706.008 to the nearest penny.*

The expected answer was £706.01, but Charles, aged 16, said that it was £706.09. His argument was that the 8 (in the .008) changed the 0 in the previous column to 9. 'The two noughts are really ten, so when I correct I make the ten go down one so that it becomes nine.' This is in effect a double error, since even if it had been correct to think of '00' as '10' he ought to have moved to 11, making the number one bigger, rather than to 9 which made it one smaller.

(ii) *Correct £32.896 to the nearest penny.*

The expected answer was £32.90, but the answer given by Tom, aged 16, was £32.18. He said that the six in the third decimal place made the nine go up one so that it became ten; thus 10 + 8 = 18.

Much practice is necessary in correcting numbers and considering place value. If a pupil is able to estimate what is approximately the right answer, then if he presses a wrong button on the calculator he will quickly see that his answer is wrong and will retrace his steps, checking each one. In the case of complicated questions the student should be encouraged to record his estimating work and then set down his accurate work alongside so that the two can be checked. Once he gets into the habit of estimating he will do so quickly, before using his calculator; and by this means major error will probably be avoided.

CONCLUDING REMARKS

Emphasis has been placed in this chapter on the relationship between teacher and pupil. This needs to be a partnership in which both are actively involved. It is understood in particular that they will talk about the pupil's difficulties and try to discover their source. This cannot be done unless both of them are fully aware of the kinds of ways in which dyslexics are liable to go wrong. To tell a pupil that he could be successful if only he were more confident, while at the same time failing to show understanding of why he finds certain tasks difficult, is likely to diminish confidence rather than bolstering it. In contrast, if teacher and pupil work together on specific skills – the understanding of equations, estimation, the use of a calculator, and the like – this will be an encouragement to the pupil to devise other compensatory strategies as they are needed. There will be less need to panic; and he may well find that he is improving not only in mathematics but in other subjects also.

REFERENCES

Joffe, L.S. (1981) 'School mathematics and dyslexia: aspects of the inter-relationship', PhD thesis, University of Aston in Birmingham.
Steeves, K.J. (1983) 'Memory as a factor in the computational efficiency of dyslexic children with high abstract reasoning ability', *Annals of Dyslexia* 33, 141–52.

Chapter 6

The use of structured materials with older pupils

T.R. Miles

STRUCTURED MATERIALS AND SYMBOLIZATION

Dienes (1960: 31) has described mathematics as 'a structure of relationships, the formal symbolism being merely a way of communicating parts of the structure from one person to another'. Shortly afterwards (1960: 31) he speaks of 'structural relationships between concepts connected with numbers'. He then says (1960: 31–2): 'The learning of mathematics I shall take to mean the apprehension of such relationships together with their symbolisation.'

This distinction between 'apprehension of relationships' and 'symbolisation' seems to me to be of crucial importance as far as dyslexics are concerned, since they are likely to have little difficulty with the first but may well have major difficulty with the second. If they have been taught merely to memorize rules for operating with symbols then they are likely to find such memorization extremely difficult; and, as a further consequence, any sense of enjoyment or excitement at the elegance and beauty of mathematics will almost certainly be missing. Again to quote Dienes (1960: 27): 'Mathematical insights are very seldom generated on blackboards.'

We owe to Dienes in particular (and also to Montessori, Cuisenaire and Stern) the recognition that these mathematical insights are most likely to arise if the pupil is encouraged to use structured materials – rods, blocks, and so on. As is well known, Dienes himself devised what he called 'Multibase Arithmetic Blocks' (Dienes 1960: 55). The purpose of this chapter is to suggest ways in which these and similar materials can be used to help older dyslexics. Since their central problem is likely to be that of relating symbols to the operations which they represent, it is good sense that they should be able to carry out the operations first, using structured materials, and only secondly be shown how to describe symbolically what they have been doing.

In what follows I shall describe my work with these materials in the standard technology of 'units', 'longs', 'flats', and 'blocks'. The 'units' which I have used have been cubes of side 1 cm; each 'long' occupies the same space as 10 'units' placed side by side; each 'flat' occupies the same space as 10 'longs' placed side by side; and a 'block' occupies the same space as 10 'flats' placed on top of each other. To indicate that the words 'units', 'longs', 'flats', and 'blocks' are being used in this specific sense I will place them in inverted commas (see also Chapter 3, note 1).

INTRODUCTION TO THE NUMBER SYSTEM

When older dyslexics, aged, say, 14 and upwards, come to me for help with their mathematics, I have sometimes found that there are some very basic points on which they have 'missed out'. Before I attempt any formal teaching I give them the chance to talk about their difficulties (just as one does in the case of literacy difficulties); and I make clear that problems with number are very common in dyslexia and that they are in fact part of the same basic limitation which has made reading and spelling difficult. It is possible, there-fore, for dyslexics to use their reasoning ability, which is often high, to compensate for those weaknesses which have so far made mathematics difficult for them. I further add that, once they have mastered the basics, they may well find the subject an exciting challenge.

The purpose of introducing structured materials is not – as it is with very young children – to give them the chance to play and hence create the conditions where they make new discoveries. It is rather to set the stage for an adult-level discussion about the number system and about symbols and symbolization. In the course of the discussion it may sometimes emerge that they are still lacking in certain basic skills, for instance the ability to tell if one number is 'larger' than another or whether subtracting from a number makes that number larger or smaller. I have found it helpful not just to explain these different points as they emerge but rather to build up the pupil's understanding step by step even when some of the steps are already familiar. Just as in teaching literacy to a dyslexic one does not simply correct spelling mistakes as they occur but calls attention in a systematic way to the different ways in which speech sounds can be represented by letters of the alphabet, so in the case of mathematics, as I explain to the pupil, it is normally advisable to start at a very basic level in order to make sure that they fully understand how the number system works and how the different operations are symbolized. Once they know the meaning of familiar symbols it need not be all that daunting a task to learn the meaning of unfamiliar ones.

It is important to make clear that the tuition is being given not because they are 'failures' or 'thickies' but simply because, through no fault of their own, their dyslexia has made certain aspects of mathematics more difficult. If this is made clear, and if it is made clear by word and gesture that one respects the pupil's intelligence, then a return to the basics of addition, and so on, need not seem childish. In just the same way many of those who teach literacy skills to older dyslexics make clear that intellectually the pupil is not at the level of 'the cat sat on the mat' but that it is useful to discuss such words if one is making a scientific study of the English spelling system. The structured materials need not be in bright colours as if they were toys; they can quite properly be regarded as scientific apparatus and should be presented as such. I have in fact often found the case that someone who has spent many years of his life experiencing *lack* of success is greatly relieved when he finds himself able to produce a series of correct answers even to sums that are very simple; and once he has learned the correct algorithm he will come to be aware that he is in a position to work out the answers to any similar sum – an awareness that will do much to boost his confidence.

It is usually helpful at the start to demonstrate, step by step, what are the skills needed for understanding how the number system works. In my own case I often start by placing on the table, say, three 'units' (or any other number between one and nine) and ask the pupil to tell me 'how many' and to write down the answer in the form of an arabic numeral, viz. '3'. (In the discussions which follow I shall, for the sake of precision, use the word 'numeral' to refer to all such figures. This should not be taken to imply that the distinction between a 'numeral' and a 'number' is necessary at this stage for the pupil). If one carries out an analysis of what this task involves it will be found to contain two elements: (i) the ability to say the correct number word ('three'), and (ii) the ability to write the correct numeral ('3').

I then add further 'units' and point out that it is possible to carry out various operations with them – adding some of them together, taking one lot away from another, putting them in a group and repeating this operation several times, and dividing a larger collection into smaller ones. The important thing for a dyslexic is to demonstrate that part of mathematics involves *doing* and that there are many different things which can be done. These include adding three 'units' to five 'units' to make eight 'units', adding four 'units' to four 'units' to make eight 'units', dividing eight 'units' into groups of four so that each group comprises two 'units', and so on. This may also be a good opportunity to explain that multiplication is repeated addition and that division is repeated subtraction.

This can then lead to the issue of notation. What I try to emphasize is that the words and symbols that we use provide an economical way of referring to these and many other operations; they therefore relate to what has been or needs to be *done*. Thus if he picks out three 'units' and adds four others he will find by counting that he has seven 'units'. The total operation can be symbolized as:

$$3 + 4 = 7$$

If there is any doubt in the pupil's mind about how to carry out the four basic operations, or how to write them down, the structured materials can be used to provide practice. Stage one is to carry out the operation (add, divide, and so on) by handling the materials; stage two is to write down what has been done. It is also important to be sure that he understands the '$=$' sign (compare Chapter 5 of this book).

I have found that the distinction between carrying out operations and symbolizing them is often reassuring. There are, of course, plenty of operations in mathematics – for instance, calculations involving fractions, decimals, square roots, and so on – which are far more complex than adding or taking away. The important point, as one should explain, is that for dyslexics the learning of new symbols takes extra time. If in the past they have failed to understand what a particular notation was telling them to do, this can now be recognized as yet another consequence of their dyslexia; it does not follow that they are 'stupid' but only that they need to go more slowly step by step. I regularly point out to them that the principle of 'doing first – notation afterwards' is of help to dyslexics in many different contexts, since there is no problem with their ability to 'do', only with their ability to acquire and reproduce symbols at speed. In this connection music provides an interesting case for comparison, since it is possible to play or listen to a splendid tune – or even to compose one – but without a suitable notation it would be impossible to communicate to others what the tune is or how it should be played. A musical score, like the symbolism of mathematics, is thus a complex form of notation for telling people what to do. Similarly written language is a notation for recording the speech sounds by means of which we communicate with each other.

With more sophisticated pupils it may be of interest to invite them to consider how one might construct alternative counting systems. For example, it would be possible, in principle, to have a system which simply consisted of the use of marks or 'tallies'. Thus instead of the symbol '5' we might write

/ / / / /

The main difficulty with such a system, however, is that we would soon run into problems if we had to deal in very large numbers. If, for instance, we needed to refer to the number 'one thousand' this would involve writing a tally mark a thousand times! This would not only be very time-consuming; it is likely also that somewhere along the line we would 'slip one' or lose count.

There is something of a palliative in the form of the 'tally check' – a procedure which some people in fact still use. They may, for instance, be going through a list and may need to record how many times a particular event has occurred. In that case they start with individual tallies, but when the event has occurred four times instead of putting a fifth tally they put a line through the existing four. After the counting is complete the end product might, for example, be:

~~++++~~   ~~++++~~   ~~++++~~

~~++++~~   ~~++++~~   //

Because counting in fives is easy very little effort is needed to determine the number involved, which in this case can be transcribed as '27'. Within the appropriate range of numbers the procedure is less laborious than using single tallies but there are similar disadvantages when the numbers become very large.

Some pupils may find it interesting to be told about the Roman notation. This involves the use of what are in effect tallies for the first three numbers, I, II, and III (and occasionally – on grandfather clocks – IIII); thereafter a number of different symbols are used – 'V' for '5', 'X' for '10', 'L' for '50', 'C' for '100', 'D' for '500' and 'M' for '1,000'. An advantage of this system is that there is no need to use more than three of the same symbol for any one number. Thus we need 'III', 'XXX', and 'CCC' for three units, tens, and hundreds; but when one more unit, ten, or hundred is added, there is the convention that a symbol to the left of another can mean that the one on the left is that much *less* than the one on the right; thus '4' is written as 'IV', '40' as 'XL', '90' as 'XC', and so on. By this means numbers up to several thousand can in principle be symbolized, and if a new symbol were invented for 5,000 it would be possible to go even higher. Long multiplication and division, however, are far easier with the Arabic notation, and the Romans would have had to devise a different notation if it had been necessary for them to deal with the very large and very small numbers that are needed in modern science.

MORE USES FOR THE NUMBER SYSTEM

One of the most ingenious devices in our present notation is the symbol '0'. In introducing it I usually say that if *all* the 'units' are taken away there are *none* left. Instead of using any of the other numerals, as we would if there were, say, four, two or one 'units' (symbolized as '4', '2', and '1'), we symbolize this situation by the use of '0'. The corresponding words are 'no' (as in the expression 'no cats in the house'), 'none' (as in 'there are none left'), and 'nought' and 'zero', which are the spoken equivalents of the symbol '0'.

The zero becomes of particular importance in the case of numbers larger than 9. Thus instead of 10 separate 'units' it is possible to substitute a single 'long'. Here the symbolization represents the number of 'longs' and the number of 'units'. Then, instead of *no* 'units' additional to the 'long', one can place one, two, or more 'units' next to the 'long'; the names are 'eleven', 'twelve', 'thirteen', and so on, and the notation is '11', '12', '13', and so on. This is a more economical way of doing things than having eleven, twelve, or thirteen 'units', all of which have to be counted.

The numbers between ten and twenty are tiresome in that, when they are spoken, information about the units comes first and information about the tens comes second, whereas in the case of the twenties, the thirties, and so on, it is the other way round. It would be less complicated for dyslexics – as well as being more logical – if convention allowed us to say 'onety one', 'onety two', and so on, but unfortunately this is not the case. There are, of course, similar complications in other languages: thus in French 'dix-sept', 'dix-huit', and 'dix-neuf' are logical, as are 'vingt-deux', 'vingt-trois', and so on, but there seems no logic in 'vingt et un' (why the 'et'?) nor in 'quatrevingts', unless it be that 'huitante' would be difficult to say. If these conventions can be 'caught' (as happens in the case of the non-dyslexic native speaker) they are unlikely to present any major difficulty. In the case of a dyslexic, however, to require him to understand the number system of a foreign language is to super-impose one very difficult task upon another!

There is a further complication in that the number of 'longs' is in fact written on the left and the number of units on the right. Now since dyslexics regularly have left–right difficulties one might be tempted to try to forestall future trouble by instructing them to put the tens on the left. It is quite possible, however, to *place* the 'long' in the right place next to the 'units' and indicate simply that that is the order in which the pupil must write numerals; and if one verbalizes at all one can simply use the expression 'next to'. Only if the pupil goes wrong or shows signs of confusion should one intro-duce the words 'left' and 'right'. In that case the question of a mnemonic should of course be discussed, for instance that the 'longs' are on the same side of his body as that on which he wears his watch. This, however, seems to be one of those occasions when one should not meet trouble half way; and there is no point in saddling him with a mnemonic or with confusing references to 'left' and 'right' if he does not need them.

Once the idea of so-many 'longs' and so-many 'units' is under-stood, the structured materials can be used in the standard way to illustrate the idea of smaller and larger numbers. For instance one might start with a 'long' and lay one, two, three, and so on, 'units' next to it, after which one might ask the pupil to say the name of the corresponding number – 'eleven', 'twelve', and so on. The procedure can then be repeated with two 'longs', three 'longs', and so on, with the pupil saying 'twenty-one', 'thirty-seven', and so on, and writing the corresponding numerals until he understands the significance of all numbers work between 0 and 100. It is also a wise precaution in the case of the written numerals to ask him, 'Which number is larger?' and 'Which number is smaller?', and to allow him, if he is in any doubt, to check against the numbers of 'longs' and 'units'. Of course once the basic principle has been grasped it becomes tedious if one carries on exercises of this kind for too long; and instead of asking the same kind of question many times over it may be preferable simply to remind the pupil that he is now permanently in a position to represent any number between 1 and 100 both by expressing it using the structured materials and by writing it.

Next one can pass to the concept of 'trading'. By this stage the pupil will be aware that ten 'units' occupy the same space as one 'long', and he will be ready to recognize the idea that ten 'units' are *equivalent* to one 'long'. Once this word is familiar, wider generalization is possible. Thus coins can be introduced, and the pupil can be shown that use of the word .'equivalence' does not necessarily mean that the objects occupy the same space, as they do when ten 'units' are equivalent to one 'long'; the issue is whether two sets of objects are of equal value – whether one set can be exchanged or 'traded' for another. Thus a 10p piece is equivalent to ten single pence in the sense of 'having the same value', an expression which they will have already met in connection with the '=' sign and of which they can now be reminded.

The way is now prepared for the teaching of 'decomposition' – in this case the breaking down of one unit in the tens column to ten units in the units column. A familiar example is that of giving change. Thus if John goes into a shop and buys something worth 16p and hands over two 10p coins he has to be given change. From what has gone before the pupil will be aware that instead of a 10p coin John could have handed over ten single pence. It is plain, however, that if 16p is needed in all a 10p piece and six single pence will be sufficient, and John will therefore have four single pence left. The pupil can then be asked to write down in numerical form what has been happening. The number of 10p pieces is written on the left, the number of single pence on the right, just as was done with 'longs' and 'units'. What John handed over was two 10p coins and no 1p coins; the correct notation is therefore '20p'. The next task is to work out what is left in the case of an object costing 16p. Clearly what we need to know is the *difference* between 20 and 16. We therefore write what we are doing in the form of a 'take-away' sum:

$$
\begin{array}{r}
20 \\
-16 \\
\hline
\end{array}
$$

Now it is very easy to take for granted that at this point no further explanation is needed – and in the case of non-dyslexics this may well be right. Without any effort he is able to say: 'Six from nought – it can't be done; make it six from ten, which is four; change the two to a one then one minus one is none, so the answer is four.' For the dyslexic, however, life is not so easy. Quite apart from the problem, mentioned above, of having to sort out 'left' and 'right' he may wonder whether to subtract the six from the nought or vice versa, and the 'number fact' that 'ten take away six is four' may not be immediately available to him. If he has experienced the actual operation of taking away, using structured materials, he will be aware of the *reasons* for what he is doing: he will therefore be able to work out what must be subtracted from what, and if he does not have the correct 'number fact' instantly available a small amount of counting is all that is needed.

The next stage is to show him that ten 'longs' occupy the same space as one 'flat'. This is simply a logical extension of what he has been doing. The words for the numbers are 'one hundred', 'two hundred', and so on; and he is unlikely to have any difficulty in replying with the correct number if he is given, say, three 'flats', five 'longs', and six 'units'. Similarly ten 'longs' can be traded for one 'flat'. As far as the notation is concerned, what is needed is an extra column; this enables us to record, from left to right, the number of 'flats', the number of 'longs', and the number of 'units'. It is important at this point to call his attention to the notation for writing numbers such as a hundred and seven, which involve one 'flat', *no* 'longs' and seven 'units'. Once he understands the function of the symbol '0' there will be no danger of his writing a hundred and seven as '1,007'.

Similarly 'one thousand' is represented by a 'block', 'two thousand' by two blocks, and so on. It can then be seen that 'two thousand three hundred and fifty-four' could be set out as two 'blocks', three 'flats', five 'longs', and four 'units'. As a check on whether he has understood what is happening the pupil could be asked to set out the number 'a thousand and one' and then, as a difficult challenge, to write it down.

ALGEBRA

The same groundwork can also be used in introducing the pupil to algebra. Thus, to return to John and his purchase costing 16p, one might redescribe the situation as:

$$20 - 16 = \text{what? or What} = 20 - 16?$$

It can then be explained that we sometimes need symbols which in effect mean 'whatever number it is', without a particular number being specified. For this purpose we commonly use the symbol 'x'. Thus we might write:

$$x = 20 - 16$$

It can also be explained that if we need two different 'unknowns' it is conventional to introduce 'y' as well as 'x'. Other letters are also used sometimes – common pairs being 'a' and 'b', 'p' and 'q', and 'm' and 'n'. It is probably wise to introduce these new symbols gradually and perhaps even to encourage the pupil to choose the one which he prefers.

It may also help if one points out that some symbols have more than one function. For example one use for the letters 'a' and 'b' is to represent the sounds of speech, but their function in algebra is different and their function in musical notation (where capital letters are used) is different yet again.

Some pupils may find it interesting if one discusses the job done by the word 'any'. This word behaves, in effect, like a kind of blank space. The pupil will already have learned – at least implicitly – that a number word such as 'four' can apply to *any* collection of four objects. One can therefore write a '4', followed by a blank space, and this space can then be filled in as 'four tennis balls', 'four bars of chocolate', and so on. We next have to consider the situation where the blank space has to be filled by a number, for example in the sentence, 'Give me _____ apples.' In place of the blank space we can write *any* number, whether 'three', 'five', or any other. In algebra, in place of the blank space, it is conventional to use letters of the alphabet such as 'x' and 'y', but the principle is the same. There is also a link with the English word 'whatever', since the blank or the 'x' signify '*whatever* number you choose to insert'. If necessary the pupil can be reminded of the same point when he comes to do geometry and trigonometry, where the symbol θ means 'the size of the angle *whatever* size that may be'. It should also be made clear that symbols such as 'x' and 'θ' retain the same value within the context of a given problem but that if there is a second problem they will almost certainly not have the same value as they had in the first problem. It is therefore important that the pupil should be completely clear where one sum has ended and the next one has begun. In a sense, of course, it is misleading to think of x as *any* number, since it is no different from 1, 2, 3, and so on, in having a definite value; the point is rather that until we have done some calculation we may not know what that value is.

INDICES

It is also possible to use structured materials for the teaching of indices. Again one can start with a spatial demonstration: the pupil can be asked to think of a 'long' as the side of a field and then to imagine that it is a square field. It will then be clear that a hundred 'units' take up the same space as ten 'longs' or as one 'flat'. This, too, can be expressed in symbolism:

$$1 \times 100 = 100 \text{ (this refers to the hundred 'units')}$$
$$10 \times 10 = 100 \text{ (this refers to the ten 'longs')}$$
$$100 \times 1 = 100 \text{ (this refers to the one 'flat')}$$

It is of course important to give the pupil time to absorb this notation and to check that he has understood it. If he has, then the teacher can say – encouragingly, as a challenge, but not minimizing the difficulty – 'You are now ready to understand a new symbol – one which we write not *on* the line but just above it.' It can then be explained that the following expressions are equivalent: 10×10 (written), 10^2 (written), 'ten squared' (spoken) and 'ten to the power of two' (spoken). When this has been made clear, the pupil can be presented with one of the written versions and asked for the spoken version, or be given the spoken version and asked to write down one or both of the written versions.

Similarly other numbers besides 10 can have squares. Structured materials can again demonstrate this. Thus there might be a square each side of which was 2 'units', in which case 4 'units' are needed to make it up. The appropriate notations are:

$$2 \times 2 = 4$$

or

$$2^2 = 4$$

Similarly the same holds of:

$$3 \times 3 = 9$$

and

$$3^2 = 9$$

and indeed will hold of any number.

When the notion of a number's 'square' has been grasped one can pass on to the notion of its 'cube'. This, too, can be represented spatially by means of structured materials. What we call 'two cubed' requires 8 'units' and what we call 'three cubed' requires 27 'units' (or 2 'longs' and 7 'units'). The notations are:

$$2 \times 2 \times 2 = 8$$

and

$$2^3 = 8$$

and

$$3 \times 3 \times 3 = 27$$

and

$$3^3 = 27$$

At a suitable point it can be explained that the small 2 or the small 3 above a number is called an 'index' figure and that index figures can be of any size. Thus:

$$10^1 = 10$$
$$10^2 = 100$$
$$10^3 = 1,000$$
$$10^4 = 10,000$$

and so on. Although a number 'squared' is a good way to lead in to the notion of an index figure, it is important to give the pupil a variety of experiences; otherwise he may make incorrect (and some-times restricted) generalizations, for example, that an index figure is a 'little 2'.

Once indices are understood it can be pointed out how economi-cally one can refer to very high numbers. Thus although 'a hundred million' can in principle be written as 100,000,000 it is very much easier to write it as 10^8.

The next stage is to explore some further properties of indices. The pupil will already know that ten is ten to the power of one, that a hundred is ten to the power of two, and that ten times a hundred is a thousand. We may therefore write:

$$10^1 \times 10^2 = 1,000$$

Now this is 10^3 or 10^{1+2}. In other words, in order to multiply we have *added* the index figures. Similarly:

$$10^3 \div 10^2 = 10^1 = 10$$

But 10^1 is the same as 10^{3-2}; this in dividing we have *subtracted* one index figure from the other.

Now this is true not merely of the index figures 3, 2, and 1, but of any other index figure and any other base. Thus if we use the symbol 'a' for the base, and the symbols 'm' and 'n' for the indices, it is true in general that:

$$a^m \times a^n = a^{m+n}$$

and

$$a^m \div a^n = a^{m-n}$$

Once this point is clear it can be seen that there is a reason for the apparently puzzling statement that:

$$10^0 = 1$$

The pattern shown above, in which the successive powers of 10 were shown, can now be added to. As we move in an upwards direction we read 10^4, 10^3, 10^2, 10^1. If we move one more step in the same direction the pattern will look like this:

$$10^0 = 1$$
$$10^1 = 10$$
$$10^2 = 100$$
$$10^3 = 1,000$$
$$10^4 = 10,000$$

It can also be made clear that these considerations do not apply only to the number 10. Any number to the power of nought is one, or, in symbols:

$$x^0 = 1$$

Now an interesting consequence of this is that in the case of numbers below one the index figure has to be negative. This point, too, can be linked to things with which the pupil is already familiar. He can be reminded of his knowledge of fractions and decimals, and in particular that, since ten 'units' make up a 'long', a 'unit' is one-tenth, or 0.1, of a 'long'. It will not be difficult for him to think of a 'unit' being itself divisible into ten parts; and if a 'long' (equivalent to 10 'units') had to be divided into a hundred parts each part would then have to be one-tenth of a 'unit' in length. Similarly a 'flat' might be divided into a thousand parts, and again each part would have to be one tenth of a 'unit' in length. Since division is represented by subtraction of indices these operations can be symbolized as follows:

$$100 \div 10 = 10 \text{ or } 10^{2-1} \text{ or } 10^1$$
$$10 \div 10 = 1 \text{ or } 10^{1-1} \text{ or } 10^0$$
$$1 \div 10 = 0.1 \text{ or } 10^{0-1} \text{ or } 10^{-1}$$

Thus ten to the power of minus one is one tenth, and in general 10^{-x} is equal to:

$$\frac{1}{10^x}$$

Just as the index notation was seen to be helpful in the case of very high numbers, so also it can be helpful in the case of very low numbers. It is easier to write:

$$10^{-6}$$

than to write:

$$\frac{1}{1,000,000}$$

There can now be a further addition to our table showing the successive powers of ten. After 3, 2, 1, and nought the next number in the series must clearly be −1. The table – which can be extended as far as one wishes in either direction – now looks like this:

$$10^{-1} = 0.1$$
$$10^0 = 1.0$$
$$10^1 = 10.0$$
$$10^2 = 100.0$$
$$10^3 = 1,000.0$$
$$10^4 = 10,000.0$$

It is important to bear in mind that Dienes referred to his materials as 'multibase'; and although for many of us the important objective in the first place is to help pupils with base 10, it would be possible, if we wished, to construct materials in which the 'units', 'longs', 'flats', and 'blocks' represented a different base; for example, if we wished, like Dienes, to introduce the pupil to base 4 we would need to make a 'long' the same size as four 'units' and a 'flat' the same size as four 'longs'. Whether we do so will of course depend on what a particular pupil needs or would find interesting.

CONCLUDING REMARKS

Dyslexics are better at 'doing' than at 'naming', and a foundation of 'doing' is essential. The great advantage of structured materials is that they ensure that 'doing' comes first and 'naming' afterwards. If the order were reversed, as, sadly, it sometimes is in existing practice, one is in effect confronting the dyslexic with a mass of bewildering symbols and technical terms while not letting him have any very clear idea of what he is supposed to do with them. Once the necessary foundations have been acquired by 'doing', however, then the abstract reasoning, the generalizations, and the discoveries – which, after all, constitute the really exciting parts of mathematics – need present him with no problem.

REFERENCE

Dienes, Z.P. (1960) *Building Up Mathematics*, London, Hutchinson Educational.

Chapter 7

The use of patterns

S.J. Chinn and J.R. Ashcroft

A mathematician, like a painter or a poet, is a master of patterns.
(Hardy 1967)

INTRODUCTION

Two of the factors which hinder a dyslexic's progress in mathematics are poor immediate memory (Steeves 1983) and difficulty in learning the basic number facts, particularly the times tables (Miles 1983). In our experience of teaching dyslexics we have observed another handicapping factor, a poor ability to generalize and classify facts and rules in mathematics.

In this chapter we consider some of the strategies which can be used to overcome dyslexics' learning problems. These problems are, of course, exacerbated by the same lack of organization dyslexics bring to so many other areas of their lives (Smith 1978).

In our experiences of teaching arithmetic to dyslexics, we have noticed that many of our students view mathematics (which includes arithmetic, and extends into geometry, algebra, calculus, and more) as an amorphous, disjointed mixture of facts, rules and methods. Although they can understand these parts in isolation, they frequently have difficulty in mastering the interrelationships and cross-generalizations.

Our experiences lead us to believe that dyslexics need help in extending generalizations from limited areas to these interrelationships and cross-generalizations. It is one of the benefits of mathematics that rules and operations have widespread applicability and rarely, if ever, have exceptions.

A teaching scheme must acknowledge the problems of the

learner, but must not compromise the structure and integrity of mathematics. We are wary of teaching gimmicks which have limited applicability and which add little, if anything, to the developing of an understanding of numbers. For example, we understand and accept that most dyslexics have great difficulty in learning the times tables. Rote learning, finger exercises, even the powerful ARROW technique (Lane and Chinn 1986) are of dubious long-term benefit for many dyslexics. Strategies based on developing a sound understanding of number and the form and structure of mathematics are ultimately more effective and efficient, have wider applicability and are longer lasting.

In this chapter we advocate the use of patterns, not as the sole teaching method, but as an approach to the subject which is logical and therefore emphasizes the structure of mathematics and streamlines the learning of facts. The patterns are to be used as a supporting technique additional to those regularly used by teachers.

Some dyslexics develop their own strategies to bypass memory problems, but these are not always consistent. For example, Mike, a 13-year-old dyslexic, was quite successful in mathematics at school. On the Wide Range Achievement Test (Jastak and Jastak 1978) he scored at chronological age. In the subsequent oral interview he was asked to explain how he worked out some basic addition facts:

Q. How do you add 9 and 8?

The answer 17 was supplied very quickly. The method was to calculate via two 8s plus 1.

Q. How do you add 9 and 6?

The answer 15 was again supplied quickly. This time the method was based on the 3× table, using the sequence 9 . . 12 . . 15.

Q. How do you add 9 and 4?

The answer was obtained by taking a 1 from the 4 and adding it to the 9 to make 10; the remaining 3 was then added on to the 10 (easily) to make 13.

Mike's strategies were unique to each of the numbers which he added on to 9. The strategies ignored any pattern based on 9. For example, once it has been established that 9 is one less than 10, and the pattern of adding to 10 is also established, then the idea of 'taking' 1 each time to make the 9 into 10 gives a pattern. This may also be viewed as a complementary pattern to adding to 10 – but 1 less.

The idea may be extended beyond the adding of 1, 2, 3, and so on, to 9. Other series can be established, such as one which involves adding 7 to numbers ending in 9:

$$9 + 7 = 16 \text{ (one less than } 10 + 7)$$
$$19 + 7 = 26$$
$$29 + 7 = 36$$
$$39 + 7 = 46$$
$$49 + 7 = 56 \text{ etc.}$$

By using this technique, one fact, developed into a pattern, produces an infinite number of facts. The generalization is that when 7 is added to any number ending in 9, the last digit becomes a 6, and the 10s digit goes up by 1.

Patterns can be seen as sequences. Such sequences can lead to small step, success-oriented, solutions to problems. They also provide a logical momentum (that is, the pattern will carry the student forward) to facts and concepts, making them easier to teach and learn.

For example, consider the question −3 −1, to which the incorrect answers +4 or −2 are often given. A number line puts the numbers in sequence:

```
----------------> +
−5  −4  −3  −2  −1  0  1  2  3  4  5
```

An opposite presentation puts the numbers in decreasing order:

```
----------------------> −
 5  4  3  2  1  0  −1  −2  −3  −4  −5
```

This sequence and an understanding of minus relative to the sequence (which can be part of the lesson) leads to the answer −4. The sequence can be extended to provide the answer to similar problems such as −7 −6.

The use of patterns can help provide a structure and organization in mathematics, reducing the load on memory, helping understanding and helping to develop concepts. Patterns provide motivation, since success is more likely as the logical momentum of the pattern leads the learner to the correct answer.

Basic requirements; some facts which must be learnt

Although it is realistic to accept that dyslexics will have great problems in trying to learn the basic facts of mathematics, there are a minimum number of facts which are important to learn. The facts selected are the most 'cost effective', which means they can be extended to help with the learning or computing of many other facts. Two collections of facts and one concept are essential. They can be extended with efficient strategies, strategies which will also help in building a concept of number.

Collection of facts 1

The pupil needs to know the basic addition facts from 0 to 9. These will help the child learn and understand, for example, the fiveness of 5: its relationship to other single digit numbers, its position half way to 10, its breakdown to $1 + 4, 2 + 3, 3 + 2, 4 + 1, 5 + 0$ and $0 + 5$, and the way it can look:

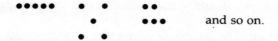 and so on.

The child needs to develop a total familiarity with 5 in all its forms, for example, five, V, IIIII, and so on.

Collection of facts 2

The number bonds to 10 are especially important for extension work, for example adding on to 9, or adding 8 to 16 as $16 + 4 + 4$. Again total familiarity is needed.

Concept

In addition the pupil needs to develop an understanding of the place values of units, tens and hundreds. (The methods to be used to teach this are not described here, but should be multisensory and involve as many manipulative materials as is possible. The teacher should note the warning given later about the transfer from concrete to abstract.)

From these starting points we can develop strategies such as the pattern of adding to 9 or adding using doubles:

$$5 + 6 = 5 + 5 + 1 \quad 7 + 6 = 7 + 3 + 3 \; or \; 7 + 6 = 5 + 5 + 2 + 1$$

Concrete manipulatives can be used to work on these facts, in other words materials such as dominoes, playing cards, money, counters, Cuisenaire rods, and so on. What is most important is that the connection between these materials and the numbers they represent is constantly taught and reinforced. The concrete example and the abstract symbol must be linked in every lesson.

PATTERNS IN NUMERACY – NAVIGATION THROUGH THE NUMBERS

With what scheme of presentation should dyslexics be encouraged to visualize the numbers from 1 to 100?

(i) The scheme should help organization.
(ii) The scheme should be consistent over all the numbers – all the numbers should be present in logical positions.
(iii) The scheme should unify all aspects of numeracy.
(iv) From the scheme should grow naturally the required extra algorithms.
(v) The scheme should be capable of supporting all future work.

The way numeracy is conventionally presented is reminiscent of a railway station run by two companies – the Addition Company and the Multiplication Company. Each has its own grid of lines, but although they coincide in some places no attempt is made to co-ordinate between them. The companies have (sometimes neglected) departments called Subtraction and Division, which generally have to use the same lines, backwards, without the benefits of signals to help them. The Addition Company has a department called Counting, which uses lines to make very slow progress.

By contrast we seek to show numeracy as a continuum, wherein Counting, Addition, Subtraction, Multiplication and Division grow from one another according to a structure (Figure 7.1).

This structure gives support to any students, including probably the majority of dyslexics, who have unique, idiosyncratic and piece-meal understanding of numeracy. Students have been encountered, for example, who see $9 + 3 = 12$ not as an addition fact but as part of the (easy for them to remember) three times table. Perhaps more important, therefore, even than its advantages for teaching numeracy from the start, is the capacity of the structure to absorb

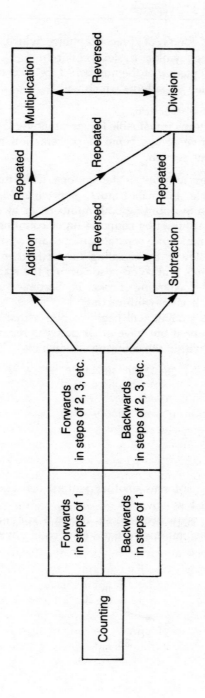

Figure 7.1 The numeracy continuum

and rationalize all kinds of preconceptions which have been brought to the subject by older dyslexic children.

We suggest that a picture of the numbers 1 to 100 should be built up from a combination of patterns which will:

(i)   confirm the above structure,
(ii) reveal other patterns (invaluable for streamlining learning), and
(iii) allow us to arrive at a scheme of presentation meeting our objectives for this section.

Students first learn to count in steps of one. Unfortunately some dyslexics are unable to make much subsequent progress in numeracy. (They add by counting both numbers, or by counting on from the first; they subtract by counting on or counting back; they divide by counting marks into separate groups, and so on.) Progress can be improved, slowly, by counting forwards then backwards with steps of 2, then 3, and so on, also varying the starting points. Almost subliminally, counting forwards becomes adding and counting backwards becomes subtracting.

Furthermore, the student will begin to notice that the number sequences being counted out have other patterns repeating within them. For example, within the counting 4 sequence,

   4, 8, 12, 16, 20, 24, 28, 32, 36, 40, 44, 48, 52, 56, 60 . . . .

it can be seen that:

   $$8 + 4 = 12$$
   $$28 + 4 = 32$$
   $$48 + 4 = 52$$
   etc.

This confirms and reinforces another pattern consequent on the properties of adding 10s.

If these counting sequences are set out in a spiral manner, the periodic nature of the patterns becomes even more obvious:

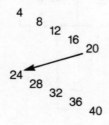

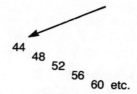

44
  48
    52
      56
        60 etc.

The counting 4 spiral can have different starting points, but only the first four are required to include every possible number. These are shown in Figure 7.2, followed by the spirals for 5 and 8 as further examples (see Figures 7.3, 7.4). Of these examples, the spirals for 5 repeat most rapidly, producing simple patterns which later render the 5× table easy to learn.

The periodic nature of addition and subtraction shown in the number spiral presentation can be exploited to reduce the quantity of extra algorithms needed. In some instances it may be possible for students to transform them into mental processes, performed with increasing rapidity, and even reaching an automatic level.

Example (i):

because	$8 + 6 = 14$
then it can be understood that	$48 + 6 = 54$
and some will understand that	$48 + 36 = 54 + 30 = 84$

Example (ii): some students might prefer to avoid decomposition or equal addition methods for $85 - 37$, as follows:

because $85 - 7 = 78$
$85 - 37 = 78 - 30 = 48$

In other instances, a more rational use of an algorithm may emerge:

Example (iii): How much more satisfying to see:

$$\begin{array}{r} 1\,2\,5 \\ -\ 7\,3 \\ \hline 5\,2 \end{array} \quad \text{rather than} \quad \begin{array}{r} \not{0}\,{}^{1}2\,5 \\ -\ 7\,3 \\ \hline 0\,5\,2 \end{array}$$

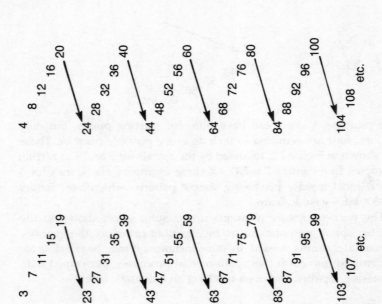

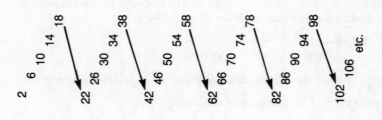

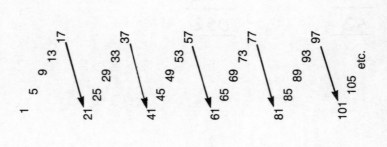

Figure 7.2 Number spirals for 4

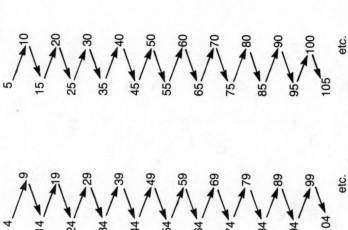

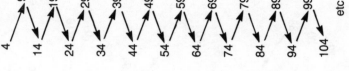

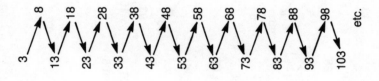

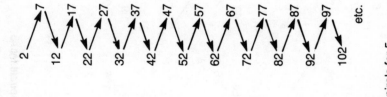

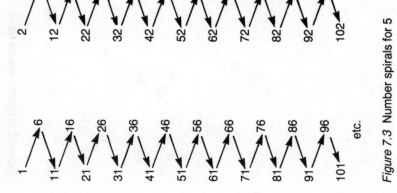

Figure 7.3 Number spirals for 5

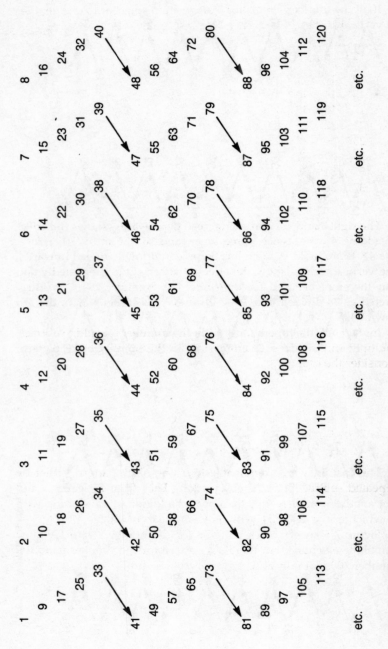

Figure 7.4 Number spirals for 8

If all the number spirals for 4 are written adjacent to one another in vertical strings, they form a block pattern:

1	2	3	4
5	6	7	8
9	10	11	12
13	14	15	16
17	18	19	20
21	22	23	24
25	26	27	28
29	30	31	32
33	34	35	36
37	38	39	40
etc.			

The right-hand vertical string, read downwards, shows the effect of adding 4 once, twice, three times, and so on, and is, therefore, the 4× times table. Adding has become multiplying. Read upwards, the vertical strings show the effect of subtracting 4 repeatedly and can therefore be used for divisions. For example, 28 ÷ 4 (interpreted as 28 divided into 4s) is given as 7, because 28 is in the 7th row of 4s.

In fact all the operations with the number 4 (add, subtract, multiply and divide) are summarized in the number block pattern. Consider the examples:

$$13 + 4 = 17$$
$$19 - 4 = 15$$
$$3 \times 4 = 12$$
$$28 \div 4 = 7$$
$$27 \div 4 = 6 \text{ remainder } 3$$

This last answer is obtainable from the block pattern, either by repeated subtraction, whereby working back from 27 leaves 3 and not another complete 4 or by repeated addition of 4s, starting with 4, which brings us to 24, with 3 remaining to reach 27.

Figure 7.5 shows block patterns for the numbers 1 to 10. They can all be extended, but the block pattern for the 10 takes us to the number 100 naturally and completes the picture.

1

2

3

4

5

6

7

8

9

1	2	3	4	5	6	7	8	9	10
11	12	13	14	15	16	17	18	19	20
21	22	23	24	25	26	27	28	29	30
31	32	33	34	35	36	37	38	39	40
41	42	43	44	45	46	47	48	49	50
51	52	53	54	55	56	57	58	59	60
61	62	63	64	65	66	67	68	69	70
71	72	73	74	75	76	77	78	79	80
81	82	83	84	85	86	87	88	89	90
91	92	93	94	95	96	97	98	99	100

10

Figure 7.5 Number block patterns

Conclusion

We propose that the teaching of numeracy to dyslexics should be organized according to the above structure, based on the patterns shared by all the numbers from 1 to 100.

Correspondingly, we propose that students should work from or refer to a page/chart of number block patterns, rather than separate and uncoordinated addition and multiplication tables. Since the right-hand vertical string of each number block pattern constitutes a multiplication table, facts are gained rather than lost, the distributive law is still clearly demonstrated and the algorithms based upon it for longer multiplications emerge naturally.

Any subsequent addition or subtraction sequences encountered by students involving positive whole numbers will be familiar, furthermore, as extracts from number block patterns.

PATTERNS FOR PRACTICE AND AIDING THE ESTABLISHMENT OF CONCEPTS

The illustrations in this section are intended to reinforce other methods of teaching such concepts as multiplication of negative numbers and to provide alternative forms of practice. Their particular effectiveness for the dyslexic will be through showing that numbers of all kinds behave in a predictable, controllable and understandable way, be they whole numbers, decimals, negative numbers, fractions or algebraic terms.

There are other specific advantages;

1. Minimal symbolism/nomenclature

The pattern in a number sequence obviates the need for operation symbols and others, which can lead to misinterpretation and ambiguity. More responsibility is placed on the student, from whom decision making and problem solving are required.

2. Practice and understanding of the arithmetical operations

Most questions will require a combination of two operations, such as subtraction to find a difference, then addition to find the next number. Through checking, the reciprocity of pairs of operations will become more evident. Generally alternatives will be encouraged.

3. Motivational considerations

Questions set as patterns or sequences are elevated into puzzles. Because of the choice of approaches, either directional or operational, which provides alternatives and the opportunity for checking, it will usually be self evident when the right answer is obtained. The reassurance of success is invaluable.

4. Logical momentum

Patterns carry a 'logical momentum'. For numbers which follow a clear pattern it is readily accepted that the pattern will continue, forwards or backwards. Students will happily allow this logical momentum to extend patterns into areas planned by the teacher to reinforce or help establish a concept.

Addition and subtraction sequences

For example:

3, 6, 9, ___, 15, 18, 21, 24

The first step in establishing the missing number in this sequence requires the recognition that it increases to the right by adding 3 or decreases to the left by subtracting 3. This discovery can be made either explicitly with, for example, a subtraction or counting on, or implicitly through a familiarity with the numbers.

The second step is to add this 3 to 9, or subtract this 3 from 15.

Number sequences of this kind provide practice at adding and subtracting, and demonstrate the relationship between the operations and their virtual interchangeability.

Patterns with powers

The sequence 4, 16, 64, 256, 1024, and so on, produced by multiplying successively by 4, rapidly gives numbers which are too large to manage comfortably. It provides a convincing argument for a knowledge of, and a use of, index notation, after which it becomes:

$$4^1, 4^2, 4^3, 4^4, 4^5 \ldots$$

Now another pattern is observable in the powers.

Decimal number sequences

Example: 16.0, 16.2, 16.4, ___, 16.8

In this sequence, each differs from its neighbour by 0.2, or 2 in the tenths column.

Example: 2.6, 2.7, 2.8, 2.9, ___, ___, 3.2, 3.3

This sequence increases/decreases by 0.1. For those who might be tempted to write 2.10 for the next number, checking the sequence backwards gives:

$\overleftarrow{}$
2.9, 3.0, 3.1, 3.2, 3.3

This provides a check on the mistake, and points towards better understanding.

Example: 4.002, 4.001, ___, ___, 3.998, 3.997

In this sequence, the increase/decrease is 1 in the thousandths column, and the missing numbers straddle the awkward region:

4.000, 3.999

Again the check backwards contributes significantly.

Algebraic sequences

The following examples help to show how algebraic terms may and may not be combined.

Example: a + 1, a + 2, a + 3, _____, a + 5, a + 6

The correct answer in this sequence is clearly a + 4, which confirms that the number term and the a term must be kept separate.

Example: 3a + b + 1, 3a + 2b + 1, _____, 3a + 4b + 1

By obtaining 3a + 3b + 1 for the above sequence students appreciate the need to keep separate the a, b and number terms. The convention that 1b should be written as just b is also demonstrated.

Example: 5x + y + 4, 4x + y + 6, 3x + y + 8, _____, x + y + 12

Here we are decreasing by x and increasing by 2 separately.

Division by decimals between 0 and 1

After carrying out a division such as 24 ÷ 0.2, with or without a calculator, the conscientious student will check whether the answer is sensible. Most of his past experience will have shown that a number becomes smaller when divided, and the answer 120 will therefore confuse any student without a thorough understanding. The following sequence could be used instead of, or as well as, a more conventional explanation, and can be organized with or without a calculator:

$$24 \div 200 = 0.12$$
$$24 \div 20 = 1.2$$
$$24 \div 2 = 12$$
$$\text{so } 24 \div 0.2 = 120$$

Division by fractions between 0 and 1

The question 40 ÷ ½ will very often produce the incorrect answer 20. This shows that there is only a sketchy understanding of ÷ or that the required algorithm has been forgotten or rejected as seemingly too bizarre. Expediently, the question becomes transformed into 40 ÷ 2. This incorrect version is more readily understood, requires a much simpler algorithm, or can be answered from memory. Without the repetition of a large section of work, it is difficult to convince students that the correct answer is 80, since, as previously, they expect a number to become smaller when it is divided. The following sequence is convincing, and goes some way towards explaining:

$$40 \div 8 = 5$$
$$40 \div 4 = 10$$
$$40 \div 2 = 20$$
$$40 \div 1 = 40$$
$$40 \div \tfrac{1}{2} = \text{something bigger than } 40$$
$$= 80 \text{ (to fit in with the other answers)}$$
$$= \text{the number of } \tfrac{1}{2}\text{s in } 40$$

Multiplying directed numbers in pairs

Best established by as concrete an argument as possible, the rules can be summarized as follows:

LIKE signs give +
UNLIKE signs give −
or $(+a)(+b) = +ab$
   $(+a)(-b) = -ab$
   $(-a)(+b) = -ab$
   $(-a)(-b) = +ab$

Any residual lack of understanding will be exemplified by questions such as 'How can two negatives make a positive?'

The following exercise relies on the convincing first line for its effectiveness in allowing the rules to derive themselves. (Because the following questions are in sequences, so are the answers.)

Fill in the missing answers. Put a + or − in each box

$$
\left.\begin{array}{rcl}
3 \times 5 &=& 15 \\
+3 \times +4 &=& +12 \\
(+3) \times (+3) &=& +9 \\
(+3) \times (+2) &=& +6 \\
(+3) \times (+1) &=& +3 \\
(+3) \times 0 &=& 0
\end{array}\right\} \quad (+a) \times (+b) = \boxed{}\,ab
$$

$$
\left.\begin{array}{rcl}
(+3) \times (-1) &=& \\
(+3) \times (-2) &=& \\
(+3) \times (-3) &=& \\
 & & \\
(+3) \times (-4) &=& -12 \\
(+2) \times (-4) &=& -8 \\
(+1) \times (-4) &=& -4 \\
0 \times (-4) &=& 0
\end{array}\right\} \quad (+a) \times (-b) = \boxed{}\,ab
$$

$$
\left.\begin{array}{rcl}
(-1) \times (-4) &=& \\
(-2) \times (-4) &=& \\
(-3) \times (-4) &=& \\
 & & \\
(-3) \times (-4) &=& +12 \\
(-3) \times (-3) &=& +9 \\
(-3) \times (-2) &=& +6 \\
(-3) \times (-1) &=& +3 \\
(-3) \times 0 &=& 0
\end{array}\right\} \quad (-a) \times (-b) = \boxed{}\,ab
$$

$$
\left.\begin{array}{rcl}
(-3) \times (+1) &=& \\
(-3) \times (+2) &=& \\
(-3) \times (+3) &=&
\end{array}\right\} \quad (-a) \times (+b) = \boxed{}\,ab
$$

PATTERNS FOR GCSE

Most GCSE mathematics syllabuses contain a proportion of work on 'investigations'. In a large number of cases, the solutions to investigations are found by discerning the mathematical patterns beneath the surface. Certain special patterns arise naturally in many different circumstances, and it is worthwhile gaining expertise in recognizing and using them. Probably the most important are:

The even numbers 2, 4, 6, 8, 10, 12, etc.
The odd numbers 1, 3, 5, 7, 9, 11, 13, etc.
The square numbers 1, 4, 9, 16, 25, 36, etc.

The triangular numbers 1, 3, 6, 10, 15, 21, 28, etc.
The Fibonacci numbers 1, 1, 2, 3, 5, 8, 13, 21, etc.
2^n (1), 2, 4, 8, 16, 32, 64, etc.

Pascal's Triangle

```
           1   1
         1   2   1
       1   3   3   1
     1   4   6   4   1
   1   5  10  10   5   1           etc.
```

Incidentally, as well as the combinatorial numbers, Pascal's Triangle contains the preceding three sequences, along its rows and diagonals.

In general, however, most investigations will seem to have a unique pattern, and students whose curriculum has been structured to include number pattern work will benefit from their experience.

SUMMARY

In this chapter it has been our intention to show that number patterns can help the dyslexic student in important ways. By reducing the overall number of separate facts needing to be acquired and learned, they streamline the learning process. The regularity and structure they bring to the subject compensate for the student's own lack of organization, and enhance his ability to establish inter-relationships and cross-generalizations.

The help is available at all stages of development, from the level of very basic numeracy to GCSE level. At almost every stage in between, number patterns can provide alternative forms of practice to aid conceptual development. They can be used as much or as little as the teacher sees fit, the flexibility of their applicability being one of their biggest advantages.

Finally, it should be added that the benefits gained through experience with number patterns are not confined to mathematics. As a quantitative form of generalization, their recognition can be useful in other school subjects, such as the sciences or geography, and in areas of everyday life.

REFERENCES

Hardy, G.H. (1967) *A Mathematician's Apology*, Cambridge, Cambridge University Press.

Jastak, J.F. and Jastak, S. (1978) *Wide Range Achievement Test* (revised edn), Wilmington, Del., Jastak Associates.

Lane, C. and Chinn, S.J. (1986) 'Learning by self-voice echo', *Academic Therapy* 21 (4), 477–81.

Miles, T.R. (1983) *Dyslexia: The Pattern of Difficulties*, Oxford, Blackwell.

Smith, S. (1978) *No Easy Answers*, Rockville, NIMH.

Steeves, J. (1983) 'Memory as a factor in the computational efficiency of dyslexic children with high abstract reasoning ability, *Annals of Dyslexia* 33, 41–52.

Chapter 8

An overview

Elaine Miles

All the contributions in the preceding chapters have been written independently and from an individual point of view. It may be useful briefly to consider what information they collectively give us both on the balance of strengths and weaknesses that a dyslexic is likely to have in mathematics, and on the approaches which have the best potential for helping him.

Tim Miles did not find a great deal of systematic research to quote, but there is clinical evidence too. Steeves's (1983) research project is very important in that it gives clear evidence of a disparity of ability between different areas of mathematics. Some of the dyslexics in her sample were on a level with outstanding mathematically talented non-dyslexic peers on the Raven Standard Progressive Matrices Test (SPM) (Raven 1958) (a test which is widely regarded as an indicator of mathematical ability); yet on a written test of computation their scores were no higher than those of children who were functioning mathematically at grade level, that is, at an average level for their form; and they were even below this level on the Wechsler Memory Test. It seems that dyslexics can be, at best, very good indeed at recognizing patterns and relationships, particularly in those situations where spatial and visual tasks are involved; and if this is correct one would expect them to be strong not only on the SPM but (provided they have learned the necessary notations) also in geometry, transformations, set theory, and so on. Miles quotes cases of a mathematics lecturer and a physics lecturer, both dyslexic, who were able to capitalize on very high abilities of this sort to compensate for their handicaps.

He goes on to examine in detail some of the areas in which the dyslexic seems to have difficulty, adducing a variety of evidence. There are systematic experimental projects exploring dyslexics' difficulties in acquiring number facts; there is evidence from the results of the Arithmetic sub-test of the Wechsler Intelligence Scale for Children (Wechsler 1969); and there is evidence of difficulties with tables. In addition there are recorded responses to items in the Stanford-Binet intelligence test (Terman and Merrill 1960); these items involve both mathematical understanding and simple computation, and dyslexics were regularly found to be strong at the first and weak at the second. He mentions, too, the probable serious effects in mathematics of a dyslexic's known uncertainty over direction and position. Such effects are well documented in the chapters contributed by the teachers. He recommends plenty of practical work with blocks to give full understanding of the processes which the symbols are used to express.

In Chapter 2 Steve Chinn draws our attention to the importance of studying differences in the ways in which children approach mathematical problems. The two extremes of style are those of the 'grasshopper' whose approach is a global one and the 'inchworm' who proceeds steadily from one step to the next. Both are needed in the good mathematician. Yet at the present time much mathematics teaching exclusively favours the inchworm approach – an approach which many dyslexics are likely to find difficult since it requires both a good knowledge of number facts and the ability to 'hold in mind' successive items in a series of numbers. The dyslexic would perhaps fare better and his errors would be better understood if more attention were paid to his favoured style of working. Thus encouraged, and with more understanding of what mathematics is about, he might have better motivation to improve his deficient inchworm skills. Chinn does point out, however, that if the dyslexic does not have a global flair to compensate for poor inchworm skills, he is likely to be very hard to teach.

Mary Kibel's account of her discovery of what works with children who have problems with the basic algorithms of addition, subtraction, multiplication and division is so vivid as to make fascinating reading. One is, of course, reminded immediately of the theory put forward by Dienes (1964: 139) in devising his apparatus, namely, that more children could advance to the stage of symbolization if they used what he calls 'embodiment-symbols'. Dienes was concerned with the teaching of mathematics to all children in general who were failing to progress in the subject, rather than with the special needs of dyslexics as such, but it is fruitful to compare his ideas on a number of points with those of several of the contributors to this book. It is interesting, therefore, that Kibel, although she makes some of the same points as Dienes, has added another important dimension for the dyslexic by stressing the necessity to practise oral language and 'tie' this language to the processes which are being carried out manually. This kind of tying together has many similarities with the 'linkages' advocated by Gillingham and Stillman (1969) in teaching reading and spelling to dyslexics. Kibel (personal communication) has suggested that for her there is a connection here with the theory propounded by Vygotsky (1986), that the chatter with which small children accompany their actions later turns into constructive thought.

Clearly we already know from numerous research projects that the dyslexic is deficient linguistically, and in my own chapter I have tried to recount the numerous different points at which linguistic ability comes into mathematics. The dyslexic needs his linguistic skills strengthened at every turn. This applies to the teaching of mathematics, just as much as to the teaching of language skills.

With Anne Henderson's chapter the scene has shifted to the secondary school level. Here it is necessary to meet the child at the stage where he is. It seems that there can be feelings of sheer terror and hopelessness at the prospect of having to do mathematics; and for anyone teaching the subject to dyslexics it is essential both to understand this and to be willing to listen in detail to what the pupil says about his fears. More specifically, the teacher needs to study what the pupil is doing as he carries out calculations and uses algorithms and to discover the underlying pattern of his difficulties as he talks his method through. She will then be in a position to appreciate some of the ability and ingenuity that he is exercising, and she will be able to adopt a flexible way to help rather than by imposing her own rules and insisting that the pupil should do it her way. Dienes (1960: 33) makes exactly the same point, being strongly opposed to any 'superimposed patterning or structuring'. It is clearly also important to teach pupils to estimate within approximate limits what answer to expect, since this will put them in a position where they can monitor their own answers. In the course of studying her pupils' errors, Henderson came across frequent examples of confusion through the overloading of the memory and the preservation of ideas from a previous example. It is not that a particular topic cannot be mastered; it is that dyslexics need more practice and experience than non-dyslexics if they are to succeed in doing so. Dienes (1964) makes the same point, insisting that the repeated experiences need to be with different materials and variables if the mathematical generalization is to be extracted from its perceptual environment or from the particular examples met.

Evidently these pupils are suffering from some of the early inadequate understanding of fundamental operations in a base ten system which Kibel was describing, and in Chapter 6 Tim Miles has described how even in the case of older pupils he finds it advantageous to fill in these gaps using similar structural arithmetic apparatus to make his points. He even finds a use for them in explaining algebra and index figures.

Finally, Steve Chinn and Richard Ashcroft have combined to show in detail how the teaching of patterns in mathematics can overcome the problems of poor working memory and make possible the calculation – and ultimate automatization – of a wide range of number facts. The same principle is employed in teaching spelling patterns rather than isolated words. At the same time, Chinn and Ashcroft point out that it is teaching them something important about mathematics, rather than supplying gimmicks to get over isolated points of difficulty. Echoes of Dienes again! 'To structure events by considering them as part of a pattern is ... the very essence of mathematical thinking' (Dienes 1960: 32). For dyslexics these patterns have to be made explicit.

There are two points which recur throughout the book. The first is that dyslexic children need to learn initially by operating with materials; only later should they be introduced to symbols – which should then be presented as a way of recording what has been done. The second is that the different types of language used in mathematics need to be taught specifically and systematically if they are to be understood.

REFERENCES

Dienes, Z.P. (1960) *Building Up Mathematics*, London, Hutchinson Educational.

Dienes, Z.P. (1964) *The Power of Mathematics*, London, Hutchinson Educational.

Gillingham, A. and Stillman, B.E. (1969) *Remedial Training for Children with Specific Disability in Reading, Spelling, and Penmanship*, Cambridge, Mass., Educators Publishing Service.

Raven, J.C. (1958) *Standard Progressive Matrices*, London, H.K. Lewis.

Steeves, K.J. (1983) 'Memory as a factor in the computational efficiency of dyslexic children with high abstract reasoning ability', *Annals of Dyslexia* 33, 141–52.

Terman, L.M. and Merrill, M.A. (1960) *Stanford-Binet Intelligence Scale*, London, Harrap.
Vygotsky, L. (1986) *Thought and Language* (translated by A. Kozulin), Cambridge, Mass., MIT Press.
Wechsler, D. (1969) *Wechsler Intelligence Scale for Children (WISC-R)*, New York, Psychological Corporation.

Name index

Subject index